Safe Piped Water

World Health Organization titles with IWA Publishing

Water Quality: Guidelines, Standards and Health edited by Lorna Fewtrell and Jamie Bartram. (2001)

WHO Drinking Water Quality Series

Assessing Microbial Safety of Drinking Water: Improving Approaches And Methods edited by Al Dufour, Mario Snozzi, Wolfgang Koster, Jamie Bartram, Elettra Ronchi and Lorna Fewtrell. (2003)

Water Treatment and Pathogen Control: Process Efficiency in Achieving Safe Drinking Water by Mark W LeChevallier and Kwok-Keung Au. (2004)

Safe Piped Water: Managing Microbial Water Quality in Piped Distribution Systems by Richard Ainsworth. (2004)

Forthcoming
Fluoride in Drinking Water edited by K. Bailey, J. Chilton, E. Dahi, M. Lennon, P. Jackson and J. Fawell.

Arsenic in Drinking Water by WHO/World Bank/UNICEF as a cooperative effort of a series of UN agencies.

WHO Emerging Issues in Water & Infectious Disease Series

Heterotrophic Plate Counts and Drinking-water Safety: The Significance of HPCs for Water Quality and Human Health edited by J. Bartram, J. Cotruvo, M. Exner, C. Fricker, A. Glasmacher. (2003)

Pathogenic Mycobacteria in Water: A Guide to Public Health Consequences, Monitoring and Management edited by S. Pedley, J. Bartram, G. Rees, A. Dufour and J. Cotruvo. (2004)

Waterborne Zoonoses: Identification, Causes and Control edited by J.A. Cotruvo, A. Dufour, G. Rees, J. Bartram, R. Carr, D.O. Cliver, G.F. Craun, R. Fayer, and V.P.J. Gannon. (2004)

Forthcoming
Water Recreation and Disease: An Expert Review of the Plausibility of Associated Infections, their Acute Effects, Sequelae and Mortality edited by K. Pond.

For further details contact: Portland Customer Services, Commerce Way, Colchester, Essex, CO2 8HP, UK.
Tel: +44 (0) 1206 796351; Fax: +44 (0) 1206 799331; Email: sales@portland-services.com; or order online at:

www.iwapublishing.com

Safe Piped Water

Managing Microbial Water Quality in Piped Distribution Systems

Edited by
Richard Ainsworth

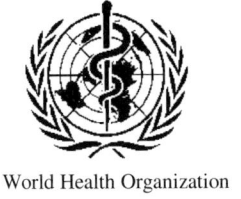

World Health Organization

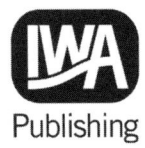

Publishing

Published on behalf of the World Health Organization by
IWA Publishing, Alliance House, 12 Caxton Street, London SW1H 0QS, UK

Telephone: +44 (0) 20 7654 5500; Fax: +44 (0) 20 7654 5555; Email: publications@iwap.co.uk
www.iwapublishing.com

First published 2004
© World Health Organization (WHO) 2004

Printed by TJ International (Ltd), Padstow, Cornwall, UK

Apart from any fair dealing for the purposes of research or private study, or criticism or review, as permitted under the UK Copyright, Designs and Patents Act (1998), no part of this publication may be reproduced, stored or transmitted in any form or by any means, without the prior permission in writing of the publisher, or, in the case of photographic reproduction, in accordance with the terms of licences issued by the Copyright Licensing Agency in the UK, or in accordance with the terms of licenses issued by the appropriate reproduction rights organization outside the UK. Enquiries concerning reproduction outside the terms stated here should be sent to IWA Publishing at the address printed above.

The publisher makes no representation, express or implied, with regard to the accuracy of the information contained in this book and cannot accept any legal responsibility or liability for errors or omissions that may be made.

Disclaimer
The opinions expressed in this publication are those of the authors and do not necessarily reflect the views or policies of the International Water Association or the World Health Organization. IWA, WHO and the editor will not accept responsibility for any loss or damage suffered by any person acting or refraining from acting upon any material contained in this publication.

In addition, the mention of specific manufacturers' products does not imply that they are endorsed or recommended in preference to others of a similar nature that are not mentioned. Errors and omissions excepted, the names of proprietary products are distinguished by initial capital letters.

The designations employed and the presentation of the material in this publication do not imply the expression of any opinion whatsoever on the part of the World Health Organization concerning the legal status of any country, territory, city or area or of its authorities, or concerning the delimitation of its frontiers or boundaries. Dotted lines on maps represent approximate border lines for which there may not yet be full agreement.

British Library Cataloguing-in-Publication Data
A CIP catalogue record for this book is available from the British Library

WHO Library Cataloguing-in-Publication Data
Safe Piped Water: Managing Microbial Water Quality in Piped Distribution Systems / edited by R. Ainsworth.
    1.Water microbiology 2.Water supply 3.Potable water - chemistry 4.Water
    quality 5.Sanitary engineering - methods 6.Knowledge, attitudes, practice
    7.Review literature I.Ainsworth, R.

ISBN 92 4 156251 X   (LC/NLM classification: QW 80)

ISBN 1 84339 039 6 (IWA Publishing)

Contents

Foreword xi
Acknowledgements xv
Acronyms and abbreviations used in the text xix

1   The microbiology of piped distribution systems and public health 1
   1.1 Introduction 1
   1.2 Waterborne disease due to contamination of the distribution
       system 3
   1.3 Microorganisms in the distribution system 5
       1.3.2   Growth of microorganisms in the distribution system 6
       1.3.3   The fate of pathogens gaining access to distribution
               systems 8
       1.3.4   Households and large building systems 9
       1.3.5   Controlling microorganisms in distribution systems 11

1.4 Traditional approaches to microbial monitoring in distribution
systems 12
    1.4.1   Regulations and guidelines for microbiological
parameters 12
    1.4.2   Principles of microbial monitoring in distribution
systems 14
1.5 Summary 15
1.6 References 15

2 Minimizing potential for changes in microbial quality of treated water 19
2.1 Introduction 19
2.2 Microbial growth factors 20
2.3 Treated water quality objectives 21
    2.3.1   Disinfection strategy and the distribution system 22
    2.3.2   Particulate content, turbidity and coagulant residual 26
    2.3.3   Organic matter 27
    2.3.4   Limiting the potential for corrosion and scale 29
2.4 Optimization of treatment 30
    2.4.1   Water sources 30
    2.4.2   Drinking-water treatment plant 31
    2.4.3   Decentralized treatment 33
2.5 Summary 33
2.6 References 34

3 Design and operation of distribution networks 38
3.1 Introduction 38
3.2 Design and operation of piped networks 39
    3.2.1   Hydraulics 39
    3.2.2   Pumps and control valves 42
    3.2.3   Access for maintenance 43
    3.2.4   Surge events 44
    3.2.5   Integrated operations 45
3.3 Design and operation of service reservoirs 46
    3.3.1   Shape and configuration 47
    3.3.2   Flow pattern 48
    3.3.3   General issues 49
3.4 Controlling disinfectant residuals by booster (relay) dosing 50
    3.4.1   Reasons for booster dosing 50
    3.4.2   Locating booster sites 51
    3.4.3   Equipment 51

	3.5	Avoiding potential problems when mixing water sources in distribution 53
		3.5.1 Modelling and planning 53
		3.5.2 Introducing a new supply 54
		3.5.3 Potential effects of mixing waters on disinfectant residual and microbial quality 55
		3.5.4 Changing flow conditions and existing deposits 56
	3.6	Potential effects of zoning networks 57
		3.6.1 Potential benefits 57
		3.6.2 Potential disadvantages 57
		3.6.3 Implementing changes 57
	3.7	Pipe materials 58
	3.8	Pipe location 59
	3.9	Protection from cross-connection and backflow at point of delivery 59
		3.9.1 Sanitary significance 59
		3.9.2 Cross-connection control 60
		3.9.3 Backflow prevention devices 62
		3.9.4 Typical property hazard ratings 63
		3.9.5 Field testing and maintenance of backflow protection devices 64
	3.10	Health related design and operations checklist 65
	3.11	Summary 67
	3.12	References 67
4	Maintenance and survey of distribution systems 69
	4.1	Introduction 69
	4.2	Maintenance and survey of reservoirs, tanks and fittings 70
		4.2.1 Sanitary significance 70
		4.2.2 Service reservoirs and tanks 71
		4.2.3 Valves and other fittings 74
	4.3	Maintenance and survey of pipes 75
		4.3.1 Sanitary significance 75
		4.3.2 Strategies for pipe networks 76
		4.3.3 Planning mains-cleaning programmes 78
		4.3.4 Monitoring effectiveness of mains cleaning 79
	4.4	Nonaggressive pipe cleaning methods 79
		4.4.1 Introduction 79
		4.4.2 Flushing 80
		4.4.3 Swabbing 81
		4.4.4 Air scouring 83

viii   Safe Piped Water

    4.5 Summary 84
    4.6 References 85

5 Precautions during construction and repairs 87
    5.1 Introduction 87
    5.2 Precautionary working practices 89
    5.3 Personnel 90
    5.4 Cleaning and disinfection procedures 91
        5.4.1 Typical cleaning and disinfection procedures 91
        5.4.2 Methods for dosing chlorine into the mains 94
        5.4.3 Practical problems 95
        5.4.4 Effectiveness of guidance for field disinfection 95
    5.5 Risk assessment and monitoring 96
    5.6 Small community-managed systems 97
    5.7 Summary 99
    5.8 References 99

6 Small animals in drinking-water distribution systems 100
    6.1 Introduction 100
    6.2 Occurrence of animals in distribution systems 102
        6.2.1 Extent 102
        6.2.2 Sampling 103
        6.2.3 Ingress 104
        6.2.4 Population size 106
    6.3 Significance of metazoan animals in drinking-water
        distribution systems 108
        6.3.1 Aesthetic problems 108
        6.3.2 Metazoan parasites 108
        6.3.3 Effect of animals on occurrence of microorganisms
               in water mains 109
        6.3.4 Association between animals and pathogens 110
        6.3.5 Protection from disinfection 110
    6.4 Remedial measures 112
        6.4.1 Range of methods 112
        6.4.2 Physical methods 112
        6.4.3 Chemical methods 113
        6.4.4 Measures suitable for different groups of animals 115
        6.4.5 Long-term control measures 117
    6.5 Summary 118
    6.6 References 119

7	Risk management for distribution systems	121
	7.1 Introduction	121
	7.2 Water safety plans	122
	7.2.1 Elements of a water safety plan	122
	7.3 Water safety plans for distribution systems	124
	7.3.1 Assemble team	124
	7.3.2 Document and describe the system	124
	7.3.3 Hazard assessment and risk characterization	125
	7.3.4 Control measures	130
	7.3.5 Monitoring to support risk management	131
	7.3.6 Verification	133
	7.3.7 Supporting programmes and management procedures	135
	7.3.8 Documentation	135
	7.5 Summary of water safety plan content	136
	7.6 References	137
Index		139

Foreword

Pressurized pipe networks provide a means for supplying drinking-water to individual dwellings, buildings and communal taps. Their widespread adoption has contributed significantly to both the reduction and control of water-related diseases. They also reduce the burden of water collection, which is borne especially by women and children, and is itself associated with much disease and injury. Further development of piped water distribution will be critical to improving health and progressing development in countries worldwide. It is no coincidence that most of our villages and towns were originally concentrated near readily available sources of fresh water such as springs, rivers and lakes.

The microbial quality of water normally changes in a piped network. Although the changes often do not have health implications, there are many documented examples of serious contamination with pathogens occurring within the piped network. When contamination occurs, it may be difficult to trace and remedy because the pipework is normally below ground and difficult to inspect.

This review looks at the factors affecting the presence and growth of microorganisms in piped networks, and the practices of water supply organizations that can directly or indirectly influence their presence and growth. The information provided is based on experience with conventional underground systems. The special requirements for systems in conveyances (ships, aircraft and trains) or within buildings are not discussed, although many of the general considerations presented here will be relevant.

The information and conclusions presented here are intended for policy-makers and those responsible for formulating water safety plans for the supply of drinking-water, as described in the third edition of the WHO *Guidelines for Drinking-water Quality* (WHO, 2004). They are also relevant to engineers and scientists responsible for water supply planning, operations and monitoring.

Many of the practices described in this review relate to the wider aspects of maintaining the fabric and integrity of the network, not just the prevention of health risks. For example, the removal of internal pipe deposits is often undertaken to increase hydraulic capacity or reduce water discolouration. Similarly, the prevention of pressure surges is normally undertaken to reduce bursts that are expensive and inconvenient to repair. However, this review shows that there are often public health reasons for adopting a more proactive approach to many of the traditional practices used in designing, operating and maintaining distribution networks.

The first six chapters address:
- the microbiology of piped distribution systems and public health;
- composition of treated waters to minimize potential for microbiological changes;
- design and operation of distribution networks;
- planned maintenance and survey of distribution systems;
- precautions during construction and repairs;
- small animals in drinking-water distribution systems.

Chapter 7 draws together this information in the context of a framework of risk assessment and risk management, adapted for application to drinking-water supply. This approach is consistent with the water safety plans described in the third edition of the WHO *Guidelines for Drinking-water Quality* (WHO, 2004).

This review is confined to distribution networks based on pressurized pipes fed by either gravity or pumps. Open-channel networks are not considered here because they provide little or no protection from contamination.

The microbial quality of water may also deteriorate in the plumbing systems of domestic and public buildings. These plumbing systems, and the service pipes connected to the supplier's distribution pipes, have the potential to greatly affect microbial and chemical quality. Plumbing systems and service pipes may not be the direct responsibility of the water supplier, and both cross-connections and backflow situations are a threat. These issues are addressed in Chapter 3. In a typical distribution system, plumbing and services account for 82% of the total pipe length and 24% of the total surface area in the system, yet contain only 1.6% of the total storage volume (Brazos, O'Connor & Abcouwer, 1986).

Therefore, the selection of service pipe and plumbing materials, and their correct installation, is important in controlling the microbial, chemical and aesthetic quality of water at the point of supply to the consumer. These issues are not covered in this review but are the subject of another text on safe plumbing practice, presently in development (see below).

This publication forms part of a series of expert reviews developed by WHO. The reviews, which are listed below, cover various aspects of microbial water quality and health.

- *Managing Water in the Home: Accelerated Health Gains from Improved Water Supply* (M Sobsey, 2002)
- *Pathogenic Mycobacteria in Water: A Guide to Public Health Consequences, Monitoring and Management* (S Pedley et al, eds, 2004)
- *Quantifying Public Health Risk in the WHO Guidelines for Drinking-water Quality: A Burden of Disease Approach* (AH Havelaar and JM Melse, 2003)
- *Water Treatment and Pathogen Control: Process Efficiency in Achieving Safe Drinking Water* (MW LeChevallier and K-K Au, eds, 2004)
- *Toxic Cyanobacteria in Water: A Guide to their Public Health Consequences, Monitoring and Management* (I Chorus and J Bartram, eds, 1999)
- *Upgrading Water Treatment Plants* (EG Wagner and RG Pinheiro, 2001)
- *Water Safety Plans* (A Davison et al., 2004).
- *Assessing Microbial Safety of Drinking Water: Improving Approaches and Methods* (A Dufour et al., 2003).

Further texts are in preparation or in revision:
- *Arsenic in Drinking-water* (in preparation)
- *Fluoride in Drinking-water* (in preparation)
- *Desalination for Safe Drinking-water Supply* (in preparation)
- *Guide to Hygiene and Sanitation in Aviation* (in revision)
- *Guide to Ship Sanitation* (in revision)
- *Health Aspects of Plumbing* (in preparation)
- *Legionella and the Prevention of Legionellosis* (in preparation)
- *Protecting Groundwaters for Health — Managing the Quality of Drinking-water Sources* (in preparation)
- *Protecting Surface Waters for Health — Managing the Quality of Drinking-water Sources* (in preparation)
- *Rapid Assessment of Drinking-water Quality: A Handbook for Implementation* (in preparation)
- *Safe Drinking-water for Travellers and Emergencies* (in preparation).

REFERENCES

Brazos BJ, O'Connor JT, Abcouwer S (1986). Kinetics of chlorine depletion and microbial growth in household plumbing systems. *Proceedings of the American Water Works Association Water Quality Tech. Conference*, Houston Texas, (Dec 8–11, 1985), Paper no. 4B-3, 239–274.

WHO (2004). *Guidelines for drinking-water quality*, 3rd ed., World Health Organization, Geneva.

Acknowledgements

The World Health Organization wishes to express its appreciation to all whose efforts made the production of this book possible. Special thanks are due to Richard Ainsworth, who acted as overall editor and provided continuity throughout the process of its development. United Kingdom Water Industry Research (UKWIR) provided financial support for the development of this review, and special thanks are due to both UKWIR and to its Director, Dr Mike Farrimond. An international group of experts provided the material for the book and undertook a process of mutual review. While authorship of individual chapters is noted on the following pages, the quality of the volume as a whole is due in large part to the review and comment provided by many individuals. The work of Paul Hunter, who provided the case studies illustrating health impacts of inadequate distribution systems or their management, is gratefully acknowledged.

Thanks are due to Ms Mary-Ann Lundby, Ms Grazia Motturi, and Ms Penny Ward, who provided secretarial and administrative support throughout the process of producing this publication; to Hilary Cadman of Biotext for editing of the text, and to all those listed in the following section for their substantive contributions to this volume.

CONTRIBUTORS

Richard Ainsworth
United Kingdom Water Industry Research, London, England.

Nicholas J. Ashbolt
University of New South Wales, Sydney, New South Wales, Australia.

Jamie Bartram
Coordinator, Water Sanitation and Health, World Health Organization, Geneva, Switzerland.

Richard Carr
Water Sanitation and Health Programme, World Health Organization, Geneva, Switzerland.

Kay Chambers
WRc plc, Swindon, England.

Joseph Cotruvo
J. Cotruvo Associates, Washington DC, United States of America (USA).

John Creasey
WRc plc, Swindon, England.

David Cunliffe
Environmental Health Branch, Department of Human Services, Adelaide, Australia.

Annette Davison
Water Futures, Sydney, Australia.

Daniel Deere
Water Futures, Sydney, Australia.

Colin Evins
Drinking water Inspectorate, London, England.

Leith Forbes
Leith Forbes & Associates Pty. Ltd., Vermont South, Victoria, Australia.

David Holt
Thames Water Utilities Ltd., Reading, England.

Guy Howard
Water, Engineering and Development Centre, Loughborough University, Loughborough, England.

Paul R. Hunter
School of Medicine, Health Policy and Practice, University of East Anglia, Norwich, England.

Mark LeChevallier
American Water Works Service Company, Voorhees, New Jersey, USA.

Yves Levi
Laboratoire Santé Publique – Environnement, Université Paris XI, Faculté de Pharmacie, Chatenay-Malabry, France.

Ray Morris
Consultant Environmental Microbiologist, Barwell, Leicestershire, England.

Francis Pamminger
Yarra Valley Water, Melbourne, Australia.

Pierre Payment
Armand-Frappier Institute, National Institute of Scientific Research, University of Quebec, Montreal, Quebec, Canada.

Will Robertson
Health Canada, Ottawa, Canada.

Melita Stevens
Melbourne Water, Melbourne, Victoria, Australia.

Michael Storey
School of Civil and Environmental Engineering, University of New South Wales, Sydney, Australia.

Dammika Vitanage
Sydney Water, Sydney, Australia.

Tony Vourtsanis
Sydney Water, Sydney, Australia.

Acronyms and abbreviations used in the text

AIDS	acquired immune deficiency syndrome
AOC	assimilable organic carbon
ATP	adenosine triphosphate
AWWA	American Water Works Association
AWWARF	AWWA Research Foundation
BDOC	biodegradable dissolved organic carbon
BFP	biofilm formation potential
CCTV	close circuit television
cfu	colony forming unit
CV	check valve
DCDA	double check detector assembly
DOC	dissolved organic carbon
GAC	granular activated carbon
GIS	geographical information system
HACCP	hazard analysis critical control point
HPC	heterotrophic plate count
ISO	International Organization for Standardization
NAS	national approval scheme

NASA	National Aeronautics and Space Administration
NTU	nephelometric turbidity unit
psi	pounds per square inch
RDOC	refractory dissolved organic carbon
RPZA	reduced pressure zone assembly
THM	trihalomethane
TOC	total organic carbon
UKWIR	United Kingdom Water Industry Research
USEPA	United States Environmental Protection Agency
UV	ultraviolet
WHO	World Health Organization
WHOPES	World Health Organization Pesticide Evaluation Scheme

1
The microbiology of piped distribution systems and public health

Pierre Payment and Will Robertson

1.1 INTRODUCTION

This chapter discusses the microbiology of piped water distribution systems and its relationship to public health. Piped systems are generally buried complex reticulations; consequently, they are relatively difficult to operate and maintain. However, they are as important as water resource and treatment facilities in ensuring the supply of safe drinking-water.

A drinking-water distribution system provides a habitat for microorganisms, which are sustained by organic and inorganic nutrients present on the pipe and in the conveyed water. A primary concern is therefore to prevent contamination from faecal material that might build up near pipes or contaminate surface or

© 2004 World Health Organization. *Safe Piped Water: Managing Microbial Water Quality in Piped Distribution Systems*. Edited by Richard Ainsworth. ISBN: 1 84339 039 6. Published by IWA Publishing, London, UK.

soil water. Generally, bacteria present in the water and on surfaces are harmless, but they are at the base of a food-chain for other free-living organisms such as fungi, protozoa, worms and crustaceans. These organisms may be present in a distribution system, even in the presence of residual disinfectant, and the water can still be free of health risks. However, excessive microbial activity can lead to deterioration in aesthetic quality (e.g. tastes, odours and discolouration) and can interfere with the methods used to monitor parameters of health significance. Therefore, additional treatment may be needed to control the quality of the treated water in a distribution system, to prevent excessive microbial growth and any associated occurrence of larger life forms (AWWA, 1999). This subject is discussed in Chapter 2, which provides guidance on operating treatment processes to minimize problems in water distribution.

Maintaining good water quality in distribution will also depend on the operation and design of the distribution system (Chapter 3), and will require maintenance and survey procedures to prevent contamination, and to remove and prevent the accumulation of internal deposits (Chapter 4). Performing any work on the system that entails contact with conveyed water or internal surfaces increases the risk of contamination. Such situations require well-documented hygienic working practices, as discussed in Chapter 5. Chapters 3–5 summarize practices to maintain microbial quality. The practices are also relevant to the prevention of problems of discoloured water, odours and tastes. The provision of tap water that is both aesthetically pleasing and safe is important, because it will discourage the consumption of alternative supplies that may not be safe, even if they appear to be so.

The traditional approach to verifying the microbial safety of piped public water supplies has relied on sampling strategies based on the end-product — that is, tap water. Guidelines or regulations describing limits for microbial content have been set by government-enacted laws in many countries and the normal rationale for these is that historical data have shown compliant water to be safe. However, the effectiveness of some of these guidelines and regulations has been challenged by epidemiological studies. Analysis of data accumulated over the 20th century has suggested that some of the microbial standards (e.g. heterotrophic plate count, total coliforms and thermotolerant coliforms) have little predictive value for public health purposes in certain situations (WHO, 2003). Outbreaks have sometimes occurred when drinking-water met such standards (Sobsey, 1989; Craun, Berger & Calderon, 1997). This is either because some pathogens are more difficult to remove or have a higher level of resistance to disinfection processes than the indicator microorganisms stipulated in the standards, or because the sampling frequency is too low to reveal contamination, particularly when it is transient.

The identification and enumeration of microorganisms is slow, and hence is not suitable for early warning or control purposes. Sampling and monitoring the

microbial quality of the water supplied to the consumer can only verify that the water was safe after it was supplied and perhaps ingested. In such situations a holistic approach to quality assurance is important and should include:
- assessment and control of source waters to prevent or reduce pathogen contamination;
- selection and operation of treatment processes to reduce pathogens to target levels;
- prevention of contamination by pathogens in the supply and distribution system.

These stages in the water supply process can be considered in the framework of a water safety plan and, where possible, the adoption of real-time controls to reduce pathogens to safe levels, from source to supply. This approach builds on the "hazard analysis and critical control point" (HACCP) system, which has gained the approval of the food industry for controlling food quality. Its application to controlling water quality in the context of a water safety plan is described in the third edition of the World Health Organization (WHO) *Guidelines for Drinking-water Quality* (WHO, 2004). Much of the information provided in this and subsequent chapters is appropriate for the development of the distribution section of such plans, and Chapter 7 provides guidance on the development of water safety plans for distribution systems.

The present chapter reviews the importance of distribution systems in supplying safe water, the fate of pathogens in such systems, and the relevance of monitoring microbiological parameters in distribution and at the point of supply for assuring water quality.

1.2 WATERBORNE DISEASE DUE TO CONTAMINATION OF THE DISTRIBUTION SYSTEM

Data from countries that have a surveillance system for waterborne diseases have provided numerous examples of the importance of a secure and well-operated distribution system in supplying safe drinking-water.

In the United States of America (USA), from 1920 to 1990, 11–18% of reported outbreaks of waterborne disease were attributable to contamination of the distribution system. From 1991 to 1996, contamination of water in the distribution system was responsible for 22% of the reported outbreaks, caused by corrosion, cross-connections, backflow, improperly protected storage or repairs to water mains and plumbing (Craun and Calderon, 1999; Craun, 1986).

In the United Kingdom, from 1911 to 1995, problems related to the distribution system accounted for 15 (36%) of 42 reported waterborne disease outbreaks in public water supplies (Hunter, 1997). Similarly, in Scandinavia, between 1975 and 1991, cross-connections or backflow were responsible for

20% of the reported waterborne disease outbreaks in community supplies and 37% of the outbreaks in private systems (Stenström, 1994).

Deteriorating water treatment facilities and distribution systems can pose a significant public health threat, as illustrated by a study in Uzbekistan (Semenza et al., 1998). More than 30% of the households with piped water lacked detectable levels of chlorine residuals in their drinking-water, despite two-stage chlorination of the source water, and were at increased risk of diarrhoea. Forty-two percent of these municipal users reported that water pressure had been intermittent within the previous two days. There was a dramatic reduction in diarrhoeal rates when home chlorination was implemented, indicating that a large proportion of diarrhoeal disease was waterborne. The authors concluded that the epidemiological data supported the hypothesis that diarrhoeal disease could be attributed to cross-contamination between the municipal water supply and sewer, due to leaky pipes and lack of water pressure.

An epidemic of cholera that began in Peru in January 1991 marked the first such epidemic in South America since the 19th century. Subsequently, over 533 000 cases and 4700 deaths have been reported from 19 countries in that continent. In Trujillo, the second largest city in Peru, the water supply was unchlorinated and water contamination was common (Swerdlow et al., 1992a; Besser et al., 1995). A water-quality study showed progressive contamination during distribution and storage in the home. Illegal cross-connections, low and intermittent water pressure and the lack of chlorination all contributed to the widespread contamination. These authors found a wide variability in chlorine concentrations in the municipal water that was distributed to dwellings. *Vibrio cholerae* was isolated from water samples. Trujillo's water and sanitation problems, which are found on all continents, reinforce the need for measures to prevent the spread of epidemic waterborne diseases at the treatment plant, in the distribution system and at the household level.

It is not only developing countries that are at risk, as illustrated by a large *Escherichia coli* O157:H7 outbreak in a small rural township in Missouri, in the USA, that had an unchlorinated water supply (Swerdlow et al., 1992b). There were 243 case patients, of whom 86 had bloody stools, 32 were hospitalised, 4 died and 2 had haemolytic uremic syndrome. In a case–control study, no food was associated with illness, but ill persons had drunk more municipal water than had the controls (Swerdlow et al., 1992b). The study showed that, during the peak of the outbreak, bloody diarrhoea was 18.2 times more likely to occur in persons living inside the city and using municipal water than in persons living outside the city and using private well water. Shortly before the peak of the outbreak, 45 water meters were replaced and two water mains ruptured. The number of new cases declined rapidly after residents were ordered to boil water and the water supply was chlorinated. This was one of the largest outbreaks of *E. coli* O157:H7 infection and the first that was shown to be transmitted by water. System-wide chlorination, as well as hyperchlorination during repairs, might have prevented the outbreak.

1.3 MICROORGANISMS IN THE DISTRIBUTION SYSTEM

1.3.1 Microorganisms entering distribution systems by surviving the treatment processes

The first barrier required to prevent microorganisms from entering drinking-water is protection of the water source. Effective water source protection, including the construction of headworks and the control of land use within the catchment or recharge area, will greatly reduce the numbers of pathogenic microorganisms in source water. This in turn reduces reliance on treatment processes to ensure water of acceptable quality. In many situations where groundwater is used, source protection measures can be designed to largely prevent contamination by pathogens.

Source protection is particularly important when dealing with small, community-managed water supplies. In many cases, community-managed distribution systems do not apply any form of treatment. Prevention of microbial entry at the start of the distribution system therefore relies on well-maintained source protection measures. Failures in source protection are likely to result in contamination of the water supply

Catchment protection has also been shown to be important in the control of pathogens in drinking-water supplies using treated surface waters (Hellard et al., 2001). Further guidance is provided in the two accompanying texts dealing with protection of groundwaters and surface waters as drinking-water sources (see Foreword).

Water leaving water treatment plants should meet stringent criteria to provide assurance that pathogens are reduced to acceptable levels. The objective is not to provide sterile water to the consumer (which is neither practicable nor beneficial). However, the bacteriological content of drinking-water leaving treatment plants should contain only very low levels of heterotrophic and aerobic spore-forming microorganisms. Low levels of these organisms indicate that the treatment and disinfection processes have been effective in removing or inactivating most pathogens. It is possible to produce drinking-water leaving the treatment plant with less than 10 colony forming units (cfu)/ml of heterotrophic microorganisms. At this level of treatment, total coliforms, thermotolerant coliforms and *E. coli* should be absent. They are much less resistant to disinfection than other heterotrophic and aerobic spore-forming microorganisms, and their presence would be an immediate indication of an unacceptable quality.

There are, however, numerous reports in the literature concerning the presence of low levels of pathogens in treated drinking-water. These occurrences usually correspond to the use of contaminated surface water sources (rivers and lakes) or to groundwater affected by contaminated surface waters. Infectious viruses have been found in treated drinking-water that meets regulations (Payment & Armon, 1989; Gerba & Rose, 1990). Oocysts of *Giardia* and *Cryptosporidium* have been found repeatedly in treated waters, but their infectivity was often undetermined and their health significance unknown.

The reasons for these findings, other than elevated source water contamination, include inefficient coagulation, inefficient filtration (e.g. failure in filtration, backwash recycling and poor maturation of filters) and poor disinfection (e.g. no free-residual disinfectant and short contact times). Pathogenic microorganisms that evade treatment and enter the distribution system may survive and be the source of an important level of endemic disease in the population (Payment et al., 1991; 1997). Therefore, the selection of appropriate processes for the removal of pathogens and the adoption of Water Safety Plan principles in operating these treatment barriers is important for safe water supply.

1.3.2 Growth of microorganisms in the distribution system

Water treatment processes are capable of reducing heterotrophic microorganisms to less than 10 cfu/ml, although waters from most treatment works typically contain higher numbers. Some viable organisms remaining in the water will multiply if nutrients are available, especially in waters that are above 15°C, and may lead to the formation of biofilms on internal surfaces. Biofilms typically contain numerous free-living heterotrophic bacteria, fungi, protozoa, nematodes and crustaceans. Older systems may contain deposits and sediments formed by the internal corrosion of metal pipes and insufficient water treatment; they may also contain many microorganisms. The multiplication of bacteria in a piped distribution system is driven by the availability of organic and inorganic nutrients in the conveyed water and in surface deposits. This subject is discussed in Chapter 2, where practical guidance is provided for the operation of treatment processes to minimize microbial growth in distribution systems.

Most microorganisms developing within the distribution network are harmless. Exceptions include *Legionella* and *Mycobacterium avium* complex, which are discussed below. There are no reports of public health problems arising from ingestion of opportunistic pathogens (e.g. *Aeromonas* and *Pseudomonas*) found in drinking-water biofilms. *Pseudomonas* and *Aeromonas* strains present in water usually do not have the same genetic pattern as those found in clinical cases during gastrointestinal infections (Havelaar et al., 1992).

Although these organisms have not been implicated in waterborne outbreaks, *Pseudomonas* has been identified as the cause of several skin infections associated with swimming pools, hot tubs and other spa facilities (WHO, 2000).

Legionella and the *M. avium* complex merit special attention. *Legionella* in a piped distribution system can grow to significant numbers in warm waters and can colonise water heaters, hot tubs, hot-water lines and shower heads. The organism is also associated with cooling towers or evaporative condensers. Special precautions need to be taken to prevent or control *Legionella* in environments such as hospitals and health care facilities, because aerosols generated by showers or spas can be a route of infection, and contamination with *Legionella* can be a significant source of nosocomial (hospital-acquired) infections. This subject is beyond the scope of this document, but a summary of knowledge and precautions is available in a companion text (*Legionella and the Prevention of Legionellosis*, see Foreword).

The *M. avium* complex is a group of bacteria that are opportunistic pathogens in man, producing symptoms similar to *M. tuberculosis* (French, Benator & Gordin, 1997; Horsburgh et al., 1994). They are ubiquitous in soil, food and water, have been found in biofilms and are quite resistant to disinfection. Strains of these microorganisms that are found in the environment have been shown to cause disease in immunocompromised patients.

Acanthamoeba and *Naegleria* are free-living amoebae (single-celled microscopic animals) found commonly in soil and water habitats. Both have been associated with water-borne infections but not through drinking. Species of *Acanthamoeba* can cause contact lens related keratitis, with the source of contamination being linked to poorly maintained lens storage cases (Stehr-Green et al., 1987). *Naegleria fowleri* is the causative agent of primary amoebic meningoencephalitis. Infection occurs after swimming or activities that cause nasal inhalation of contaminated water. *Naegleria fowleri* is typically thermophilic, growing in water up to 45° C. Although drinking-water has not been demonstrated as a source of infection, *Naegleria fowleri* has been found in distribution systems, with detection correlated with heterotrophic plate counts and the absence of free chlorine residuals (Esterman et al., 1984).

Free living amoebae such as *Acanthamoeba* and *Naegleria* can also harbour bacterial pathogens such as *Legionella* and mycobacteria, and may play a role in the survival of these organisms in drinking-water environments and in their pathogenesis (Lee & West, 1991; Steinert et al., 1998).

Bacteria present in the water and on surfaces are at the base of a food-chain for other organisms such as fungi, protozoa, worms and crustaceans. Chapter 6 discusses the occurrence and significance of metazoan (many-celled) animals in treated drinking-water distribution systems. In temperate countries, no population of pathogenic animals has been found in a distribution system. In tropical climates, the only potential health hazard that has been postulated

(WHO, 1996) arises in countries where water fleas (*Cyclops*) are the intermediate host of the guinea worm (*Dracunculus medinensis*). However, this is a theoretical risk as there is no evidence that guinea worm transmission occurs from piped drinking-water supplies. Generally, the presence of animals has largely been regarded by water suppliers as an "aesthetic" problem, either directly or through their association with discoloured water (see Chapter 6 for further discussion).

1.3.3 The fate of pathogens gaining access to distribution systems

Biofilms, sediments and corrosion products may harbour pathogenic microorganisms introduced through inefficient treatment or breaches of the integrity of the distribution system. Buried in the sediments or embedded in the biofilm, pathogens could be released during repairs and cleaning operations, or by erosion caused by sudden changes in flow patterns. Survival depends on their nature and the microbial activity in the biofilm. Only a few pathogenic bacterial species may multiply if favourable conditions, such as warm water and appropriate nutrients, are present (LeChevallier et al., 1999a; 1999b).

Viruses and protozoan parasites are obligate parasites and they need a human or animal host to multiply. If they enter the pipe network, they can only survive for a limited period; the infective dose for human hosts is likely to be reached only if large accumulations occur within system deposits. Such accumulations may occur as a result of cross-connections, backflow or contamination (see Box 1.1).

Although there are currently no reports of health effects directly attributed to the long-term survival of pathogens within a distribution system, such organisms have been shown to persist within biofilms, thereby presenting a potential underlying health concern to consumers (Szewzyk et al., 2000). Biofilms contain many sorption sites that can bind and accumulate organic and inorganic contaminants, as well as particulate and colloidal matter (Flemming, 1995). Within biofilms, microbial pathogens can be protected from biological, physical, chemical and environmental stresses, including predation, desiccation and changes or fluxes in the environment (Buswell et al., 1998; Walker et al., 1995).

Bacterial pathogens such as *Helicobacter pylori* (Mackay et al., 1998), enterotoxigenic *E. coli* (Szewzyk et al., 1994), *Salmonella typhimurium* (Armon et al. 1997) and *Campylobacter* species (Buswell et al., 1998) can persist within biofilms formed in experimental laboratory systems. The potential therefore exists for such pathogens to accumulate and persist within a municipal distribution system, although so far they have not been isolated directly from such systems. Model enteric viruses (B40-8 and MS2 bacteriophages) have also been shown to accumulate and persist within biofilms formed in the laboratory (Storey & Ashbolt, 2001), although again these organisms have not been isolated directly from a municipal water distribution system. The interaction of viruses with pipe biofilms has been neglected or ignored in the past (Ford, 1999); however, recent research has demonstrated its potential significance (Storey and Ashbolt, 2003b)

Problems may therefore arise in distribution pipe systems when clusters of biofilm-associated pathogens become detached from either substrata or biofilm matrices by physical, chemical or biological processes. Detached biomass could compromise the microbiological quality of distribution waters by providing a continual contamination of the bulk water through the release of sorbed pathogens and indicators. These mobilized pathogens, which may exist at concentrations greater than an infective dose, have the potential to reach consumers through the ingestion of contaminated water or food contaminated with such water, inhalation of aerosols or breaks in the skin (Ashbolt, 1995). For example, in a risk model that has been developed for the distribution of recycled water there is evidence to suggest that, even during normal operating conditions (1 virus per 100 l of recycled water), enteric viruses may accumulate within distribution pipe biofilms in sufficient numbers to present a risk to consumers should a biofilm slough off from the pipe (Storey & Ashbolt, 2003a). These studies support the view that preventing the accumulation of deposits and biofilms in a distribution system should be an important component of a water safety plan (see Chapter 7).

1.3.4 Households and large building systems

Water usage, pipe materials and water-purification devices (point-of-use or point-of-entry) can positively or negatively affect water quality in buildings.

Water in household or building pipes can stagnate for long periods, leading to deterioration in the microbial and chemical quality of the water. Buildings at risk include schools during a vacation period, hotels with intermittent room occupancy, large buildings relatively unoccupied during weekends and sections of hospitals closed for long periods. These situations require planning from responsible authorities to ensure public health protection.

> **Box 1.1.** Persistence of *Cryptosporidium* oocysts in distribution after an outbreak of cryptosporidiosis.
>
> During March 2000, the town of Clitheroe in Lancashire, England was affected by an outbreak of cryptosporidiosis that affected at least 58 people. Most of the cases resided in an area supplied by a single spring source. The supply provided water to 17 252 people and was chlorinated but not filtered. It rapidly became clear that the source of contamination was cattle grazing near the spring. As soon as the water source was implicated in the outbreak, the supply was switched to a much larger and better-treated supply.
>
> Of interest was the persistence of oocysts in distribution long after the source had been switched. The source was changed on the evening after the first outbreak meeting on 16 March and the system was flushed by opening fire hydrants in the town. For the following days, multiple (up to 23 per day) 10-litre samples were collected from consumers' taps. Despite the flushing, oocysts were detected in tap samples for 10 consecutive days, although in decreasing numbers. However, on 20 March there was a peak (mean 0.2 oocysts/l) following a burst main. Because of this, the public were advised on 21 March to boil all drinking-water.
>
> On 26 and 27 March, all samples were negative and it was decided to reduce the number of daily samples. However, on the following day, two of three samples were positive (mean 0.23 oocysts/l) and further samples were positive over the following few days. This increase coincided with a decision to sample from fire hydrants rather than consumers' taps.
>
> This outbreak demonstrated the importance of the distribution system, even in outbreaks due to source water contamination. The pathogen was retained in the system even after vigorous flushing. Although the epidemiological evidence suggested that nobody became infected after the change in supply, persistence of oocysts led to the boil water advice. Partly based on the increased counts in water from fire hydrant samples, the investigators suggested that oocysts were being trapped in biofilm in the distribution network and then being released back into the supply.
>
> Source: Howe et al. (2002).

The presence of properly designed and maintained water purification devices offers some level of protection to the consumer. Filters capable of removing micron-size particles or smaller can provide an effective barrier against incoming contaminated water and bacterial and parasitic pathogens. They can be used to reduce risks for vulnerable individuals (e.g. people with acquired immune deficiency syndrome (AIDS) and other immunocompromised individuals). They may also be useful in areas where water treatment and distribution are not reliable (e.g. loss of pressure, inadequate or intermittent treatment). In these cases, filtration should be followed by disinfection (e.g. chlorine or ultraviolet radiation).

Point-of-use and point-of-entry filtering devices can retain large numbers of microorganisms as well as particulate matter. Multiplication of heterotrophic bacteria is frequent in such units, but health effects have not been reported. The issue of pathogens captured in these units has been studied extensively (Geldreich & Reasoner, 1989). Although some pathogens can survive in the matrix of filters, they are usually overcome by the growth of heterotrophic bacteria that have a much higher capacity to multiply in this environment.

1.3.5 Controlling microorganisms in distribution systems

Current practice in many countries is to use disinfectant residuals to control the growth of microorganisms in distribution systems and to act as a final barrier, to help maintain the microbial safety of the water. The various options for disinfection are discussed in Chapter 2. Realistic residual concentrations only inactivate the least resistant microorganisms such as *E. coli* and the thermotolerant coliforms that are used as the main indicators of water safety (Payment, 1999). Absence of coliforms may create a false sense of security because many viral and parasitic pathogens are resistant to a low level of disinfectant. Therefore, the maintenance of a disinfectant residual or an increase in disinfectant dose should never be regarded as a substitute for the rigorous application of the operational and maintenance practices described in this review. However, the loss of chlorine residual can be used as an indicator of intrusion if an appropriate monitoring frequency is established, especially if continuous monitoring facilities are in place in the distribution system.

In some countries and in many small community-managed piped water supplies, no disinfectant residual is applied to maintain quality during distribution. In these cases, prevention of the ingress of pathogenic microorganisms must be assured, to protect water quality. This relies on regular sanitary inspection of distribution systems to identify potential leaks or parts of the system where ingress could occur. In addition, attention should be paid to areas where faecal material builds up close to the pipe and where surface or soil water would be likely to become contaminated. The results of the sanitary inspection should be used to define preventive maintenance and remedial actions (where necessary). Maintenance of water quality in nondisinfected piped-water supplies requires proper training of system operators and managers and, in the case of community-managed supplies, on-going support through surveillance.

In large systems, particularly where disinfectant residual is not maintained, nutrient levels should be controlled to reduce the potential for biofilm growth

1.4 TRADITIONAL APPROACHES TO MICROBIAL MONITORING IN DISTRIBUTION SYSTEMS

1.4.1 Regulations and guidelines for microbiological parameters

Total coliforms

Coliforms have been used extensively as a basis for regulating the microbial quality of drinking-water. Initially total coliforms were used as indicators of faecal contamination and hence of the possible presence of enteric pathogens. However, many species of bacteria in the total coliform group survive and grow in the environment, and their value as an indicator of faecal contamination has been questioned by many regulatory agencies. Strains of total coliform bacteria may colonise surfaces within systems and become part of a biofilm (Power & Nagy, 1989; LeChevallier, 1990). The environmental conditions that favour this process are water temperatures greater than 15°C, neutral pH and adequate concentrations of assimilable organic carbon (AOC). In temperate climates, growth events typically occur during the summer months, but in tropical or subtropical climates they may occur year-round.

Their ability to thrive in the environment or in a drinking-water distribution system makes total coliforms an unreliable index of faecal contamination. However, total coliforms can be used in operational monitoring as a measure of deterioration of water quality through distribution systems. Detection of these organisms can reveal microbial growth and possible biofilm formation, as well as ingress of foreign material including soil. However, heterotrophic plate counts (HPCs) detect a wider range of organisms and are generally considered better indicators for these conditions than total coliforms.

Escherichia coli and thermotolerant coliforms

Escherichia coli (*E. coli*) is the faecal indicator of choice used in WHO *Guidelines for Drinking-water Quality* (WHO, 2004) and several countries are including this organism in their regulations as the primary indicator of faecal pollution. Current data suggest that *E. coli* is almost exclusively derived from the faeces of warm-blooded animals. Its presence in drinking-water is interpreted as an indication of recent or substantial post-treatment faecal contamination or inadequate treatment. Thermotolerant coliforms include *E. coli* and also some types of *Citrobacter*, *Klebsiella* and *Enterobacter*. Although thermotolerant species other than *E. coli* can include environmental organisms, populations of thermotolerant coliforms detected in most waters are predominantly composed of *E. coli*. As a result, thermotolerant coliforms are regarded as a less reliable but acceptable indicator of faecal pollution.

In using *E. coli* or thermotolerant coliforms as an indicator of faecal pollution, a number of issues need to be considered. First, although *E. coli* does not readily grow outside the gut of warm-blooded animals in temperate regions, there is some evidence to suggest that it may grow in the natural environment in tropical regions (Byanppanahalli & Fujioka, 1998). However, in most cases, *E. coli* would be out-competed by other environmental bacteria; therefore, whether growth occurs in nature is questionable. If such growth were to be found in certain tropical regions, then regulations would have to be based upon alternative indicators of post-treatment faecal contamination in storage and distribution systems, such as intestinal enterococci and *Clostridium perfringens* spores (Ashbolt, Grabow & Snozzi, 2001).

Second, *E. coli* is extremely sensitive to disinfection (LeChevallier et al., 2003). Its presence in a water sample is a sure sign of a major deficiency in the treatment or integrity of the distribution system. However, its absence does not by itself provide sufficient assurance that the water is free of risks from microbes. Many viral and protozoan pathogens are significantly more resistant to disinfection and may survive exposure to disinfectant that inactivates *E. coli*. Ingress of sewage into a distribution system conveying water with a disinfectant residual might not be detected using *E. coli* alone: these bacteria might be inactivated while other pathogens remained viable.

Heterotrophic plate count

The HPC was among the first parameters used to monitor the microbial quality of drinking-water. Following the work of Koch in the late 1800s, HPC was used to monitor the safety of finished drinking-water. However, in recent times, HPC has become an indicator of general water quality within distribution systems (WHO, 2003).

Heterotrophic microorganisms are indigenous to water (and biofilms) and are always present in greater concentrations than coliform bacteria in distribution and storage systems. An increase in HPC indicates treatment breakthrough, post-treatment contamination, growth within the water conveyed by the distribution system or the presence of deposits and biofilms in the system. A sudden increase in HPCs above historic baseline values should trigger actions to investigate and, if necessary, remediate the situation. There is no evidence that heterotrophic microorganisms in distribution systems are responsible for public health effects in the general population through ingestion of drinking-water (WHO, 2003).

Some countries use a nonmandatory maximum HPC of 500 cfu/ml at 35°C, because concentrations greater than this interfere with the recovery of coliform bacteria by membrane filtration techniques based on lactose fermentation. However, newer coliform detection methods based on the metabolism of chromogenic substrates are not prone to this interference.

1.4.2 Principles of microbial monitoring in distribution systems

The purpose of microbial monitoring programmes in distribution systems is to ensure that water supplies comply with applicable guidelines, standards or regulations.

Guidance on methods for sampling and monitoring is part of internationally accepted documents (ISO, 1980–98). Promulgated requirements or recommendations usually appear simplistic. They are often based on population-served criteria such as *"4 samples per month, if population is less than 5000"*. Programmes based on such criteria are ineffective for monitoring the quality of the water delivered to all consumers.

In theory, microbial monitoring could be achieved by a programme of frequent monitoring at every storage reservoir and service connection throughout the system. However, such a strategy would be prohibitively expensive and could only verify that the water was safe after it was supplied, because the identification and enumeration of microorganisms is too slow to be suitable for early warning or control purposes.

One way to monitor effectively is to perform both routine sampling for microbial quality and real-time (and possibly online) monitoring of parameters linked to microbial quality at selected locations throughout the storage and distribution system. With a good knowledge of the system's hydraulics this approach can be cost-effective and can quickly provide warnings of system failures related to health risks. Potential surrogate parameters are free chlorine, water pressure, dissolved oxygen and turbidity. Sudden anomalous changes in any of these parameters may indicate a problem with the system. A monitoring programme should include directions on data interpretation and corrective actions to be taken when limits are exceeded.

The function of microbial monitoring in distribution is recognized in the water supply plans described in Chapter 7. A water safety plan for the management of distribution systems involves three types of monitoring (see Section 7.3.3):

- operational monitoring to support on-going management of the safety of the system;
- process validation for the design of treatment processes and other control measures;
- verification to check that the entire water supply system is functioning correctly.

Routine microbial monitoring normally fulfils the verification role by acting as a final check of water safety. It verifies that the system is functioning properly; it should not be relied upon for operational control.

Periodic sanitary surveys of the storage and distribution system are an important part of any water safety plan. Such surveys are inexpensive to carry out and can complement water quality measurements. They are essential for small community-managed supplies where verification of water quality may be infrequent. Chapters 4 and 7 provide guidance on sanitary surveys and routine inspections.

1.5 SUMMARY

Good quality drinking-water can suffer serious contamination in distribution systems because of breaches in the integrity of the pipework and storage reservoirs. Many outbreaks of waterborne disease have been attributed to such events.

All distribution systems harbour active populations of microorganisms that do not threaten public health. Nevertheless, in many countries it is usual to maintain a disinfectant residual to control bacterial proliferation in the body of water supplied. This will limit the development of tastes and odours produced by biofilms, and may also inactivate low levels of some pathogens that gain entry to the network. Although there are currently no reports of health effects directly attributed to the long-term survival of pathogens within a distribution system, there is a potential for such organisms to accumulate and persist within biofilms. Experimental studies confirm this potential and support the view that preventing the accumulation of deposits and biofilms in a distribution system should be an important component of a water safety plan.

The routine monitoring of microbial indicators, such as *E. coli* (or alternatively thermotolerant coliforms), can be used as part of a final check on water quality (verification). Such monitoring should not be the only method for managing risk or supporting decisions about the operation of the distribution system. Safe drinking-water is best achieved by adopting a holistic approach based on design, operational practices and maintenance procedures that takes account of biological hazards. This approach is the basis of the water safety plans described in Chapter 7. Monitoring has an important role as part of water safety plans and should include parameters that are capable of revealing both potential contamination (due to lack of system integrity) and actual contamination.

1.6 REFERENCES

Armon R et al. (1997). Survival of *Legionella pneumophila* and *Salmonella typhimurium* in biofilm systems. *Water Science and Technology*, 35(11–12):293–300.

Ashbolt N (1995). Public health water microbiology for the 21st century. In: Gilbert GL, ed., *Recent Advances in Microbiology*, vol. 3. The Australian Society for Microbiology Inc., Melbourne, 173–214.

Ashbolt NJ, Grabow WOK, Snozzi M (2001). Indicators of microbial water quality, Chap. 13. In: Fewtrell L, Bartram J, eds. *Water quality: guidelines, standards and health: risk assessment and management for water related infectious diseases*. IWA Publishing, London.

AWWA (1999). *Water quality and treatment. A handbook of community water supplies*, 5th ed. McGraw-Hill Inc, New York.

Besser RE et al. (1995). [Prevention of cholera transmission: rapid evaluation of the quality of municipal water in Trujillo, Peru.] *Boletin de la Oficina Sanitariums Panamericana*, 119(3):189–94.

Buswell CM et al. (1998). Extended survival and persistence of *Campylobacter* spp. in water and aquatic biofilms and their detection by immunofluorescent-antibody and -rRNA staining. *Applied and Environmental Microbiology*, 64(2):733–741.

Byanppanahalli MN, Fujioka RS (1998). Evidence that tropical soil can support the growth of *Escherichia coli*. *Water Science and Technology*, 38(12):171–174.

Craun GF (1986). *Waterborne diseases in the United States*. CRC Press Inc., Boca Raton, Florida, USA.

Craun GF, Berger PS, Calderon RL (1997). Coliform bacteria and waterborne disease outbreaks. *Journal of the American Water Works Association*. 89(3):96–104.

Craun GF, Calderon RL (1999). Waterborne disease outbreaks: their causes, problems, and challenges to treatment barriers. *AWWA manual M–48: waterborne pathogens*. American Water Works Association, Denver, USA.

Esterman A et al. (1984). The association of *Naegleria fowleri* with the chemical, microbiological and physical characteristics of South Australian water supplies. *Water Research*, 18:549–553.

Flemming HC (1995). Sorption sites in biofilms. *Water Science and Technology*, 32(8):27–33.

Ford TE (1999). Microbiological safety of drinking water: United States and global perspectives. *Environmental Health Perspectives*, 107(Suppl 1):191–206.

French AL, Benator DA, Gordin FM (1997). Nontuberculous mycobacterial infections. *Medical Clinics of North America*, 81(2):361–79.

Geldreich EE, Reasoner DJ (1989). Home water treatment devices and water quality. In: McFeters GA, ed. *Drinking water microbiology*. (Springer–Verlag, New York, 147–167.

Gerba CP, Rose JB (1990). Viruses in source and drinking water. Chap 18. In: McFeters GA, ed. *Drinking water microbiology: progress and recent developments*. Springer–Verlag, New York.

Havelaar AH et al. (1992). Typing of *Aeromonas* strains from patients with diarrhoea and from drinking water. *Journal of Applied Bacteriology*, 72(5):435–444.

Hellard ME et al. (2001). A randomised, blinded, controlled trial investigating the gastrointestinal health effects of drinking water quality. *Environmental Health Perspectives*, 109(8):773–778.

Horsburgh CR Jr et al. (1994). Environmental risk factors for acquisition of *Mycobacterium avium* complex in persons with human immunodeficiency virus infection. *Journal of Infectious Diseases*, 170(2):362–7.

Howe AD et al. (2002). *Cryptosporidium* oocysts in a water supply associated with an outbreak of cryptosporidiosis. *Emerging Infectious Diseases*, 8(6):619–24.

Hunter P (1997). *Waterborne disease: epidemiology and ecology*. John Wiley & Sons, Chichester, UK.

ISO 5667–1:1980 Water quality—Sampling—Part 1: Guidance on the design of sampling programmes (ISO 5667-1:1980/Cor 1:1996)

ISO 5667–2:1991 Water quality—Sampling—Part 2: Guidance on sampling techniques.

ISO 5667–3:1994 Water quality—Sampling—Part 3: Guidance on the preservation and handling of samples.

ISO 5667–4:1987 Water quality—Sampling—Part 4: Guidance on sampling from lakes, natural and man-made.

ISO 5667–5:1991 Water quality—Sampling—Part 5: Guidance on sampling of drinking water and water used for food and beverage processing.

ISO 5667–8:1993 Water quality—Sampling—Part 8: Guidance on the sampling of wet deposition.

ISO 5667–11:1993 Water quality—Sampling—Part 11: Guidance on sampling of groundwaters.

ISO 5667–14:1998 Water quality—Sampling—Part 14: Guidance on quality assurance of environmental water sampling and handling.
LeChevallier MW (1990). Coliform regrowth in drinking water: a review. *Journal of the American Water Works Association*, 82:74–86.
LeChevallier MW et al. (1999a). Committee report: emerging pathogens — bacteria. *Journal of the American Water Works Association*, 91(9):101–109.
LeChevallier MW et al. (1999b). Committee report: emerging pathogens — viruses, protozoa, and algal toxins. *Journal of the American Water Works Association*, 91(9):110–121.
LeChevallier MW et al. (2003). *Drinking-water treatment and water quality: the impact of treatment on microbial water quality and occurrence of pathogens and indicators in surface water*. WHO, Geneva and IWA Publishing, London.
Lee JV, West AA (1991). Survival and growth of *Legionella* species in the environment. *Society of Applied Bacteriology symposium series*, 20:121S–129S.
Mackay WG et al. (1998). Biofilms in drinking water systems — a possible reservoir for *Helicobacter pylori*. *Water Science and Technology*, 38(12):181–185.
Payment P (1999). Poor efficacy of residual chlorine disinfectant in drinking water to inactivate waterborne pathogens in distribution system. *Canadian Journal of Microbiology*, 45:709–715.
Payment P, Armon R (1989). Virus removal by drinking water treatment processes. *CRC Critical Reviews in Environmental Control*, 19:15–31.
Payment P et al. (1991). A randomized trial to evaluate the risk of gastrointestinal disease due to the consumption of drinking water meeting currently accepted microbiological standards. *American Journal of Public Health*, 81:703–708.
Payment P et al. (1997). A prospective epidemiological study of gastrointestinal health effects due to the consumption of drinking water. *International Journal of Environmental Health Research*, 7:5–31.
Power KN, Nagy LA (1989). *Bacterial regrowth in water supplies*. Report No. 4, Urban Water Research Association of Australia.
Semenza JC et al. (1998). Water distribution system and diarrheal disease transmission: a case study in Uzbekistan. *American Journal of Tropical Medicine and Hygiene*, 59(6):941–6.
Sobsey MD (1989). Inactivation of health related microorganisms in water by disinfection processes. *Water Science and Technology*, 21(3):179–195.
Stehr-Green JK et al. (1987). *Acanthamoeba* keratitis in soft contact lens wearers. A case control study. *Journal of the American Medical Association*, 258:57–60.
Steinert M et al. (1998). *Mycobacterium avium* bacilli grow saprozoically in coculture with *Acanthamoeba polyphaga* and survive within cyst walls. *Applied and Environmental Microbiology*, 64:2256–2261.
Stenström TA (1994). A review of waterborne outbreaks of gastroenteritis in Scandinavia. In: Golding AMB et al., eds. *Water and Public Health*. Smith-Gordon & Co., London, UK.
Storey MV, Ashbolt NJ (2001). Persistence of two model enteric viruses (B40-8 and MS2 bacteriophages) in water distribution pipe biofilms. *Water Science and Technology*, 43(12):133–138.
Storey MV, Ashbolt NJ (2003a). A risk model for enteric virus accumulation and release from recycled water distribution pipe biofilms. *Water Science and Technology. Water Supply*, 3(3):93–100.
Storey MV, Ashbolt NJ (2003b). Enteric virions and microbial biofilms — an additional source of public health concern? *Water Science and Technology*, 48(3):97–104.
Swerdlow DL et al. (1992a). Waterborne transmission of epidemic cholera in Trujillo, Peru: lessons for a continent at risk. *Lancet*, 340(8810):28–33

Swerdlow DL et al. (1992b). A waterborne outbreak in Missouri of *Escherichia coli* O157:H7 associated with bloody diarrhea and death. *Annals of Internal Medicine*, 117(10):812–9.

Szewzyk U et al. (1994). Growth and *in situ* detection of a pathogenic *Escherichia coli* in biofilms of a heterotrophic water-bacterium by use of 16S- and 23S-rRNA directed fluorescent oligonucleotide probes. *FEMS Microbiology Ecology*, 13:169–176.

Szewzyk U et al. (2000). Microbiological safety of drinking water [review]. *Annual Review of Microbiology*, 54:81-127.

Walker JT et al. (1995). Heterogeneous mosaic biofilm — a haven for waterborne pathogens. In: Costerton JW & Lappin-Scott HM, eds. *Microbial biofilms*. University Press, Cambridge, 196–204.

WHO (1996) *Guidelines for drinking-water quality*, 2nd ed., vol. 2. *Health criteria and other supporting information*. World Health Organization, Geneva, 68–70.

WHO (2000) *Guidelines for safe recreational waters*, vol. 2. *Swimming pools, spas and similar recreational-water environments.* World Health Organization, Geneva (In process of finalization).

WHO (2003) *Heterotrophic plate counts and drinking-water safety: the significance of HPCs for water quality and human health.* Eds Bartram J, Cotruvo J, Exner M, Fricker C, Glasmacher A. World Health Organization, Geneva, IWA Publishing.

WHO (2004) *Guidelines for drinking-water quality*, 3rd ed., World Health Organization, Geneva.

2
Minimizing potential for changes in microbial quality of treated water

Yves Levi

2.1 INTRODUCTION

The microbial quality of drinking-water can change as it travels from the treatment plant to the extremities of the distribution network. Microbial proliferation will depend on the:
- transit times
- system condition
- construction materials
- water temperature
- disinfectant residual
- hydraulic conditions
- initial physical, chemical and microbial characteristics of the treated water.

© 2004 World Health Organization. *Safe Piped Water: Managing Microbial Water Quality in Piped Distribution Systems*. Edited by Richard Ainsworth. ISBN: 1 84339 039 6. Published by IWA Publishing, London, UK.

It is not meaningful or practicable to strive for a sterile drinking-water network devoid of all microorganisms. The principal objective is to remove pathogenic organisms from the water supply and prevent contamination during distribution. This requires effective management of the operation, maintenance and cleanliness of the distribution network. The management process should include optimization of treatment to minimize the entry of microbial nutrients and deposit-forming components into the network. This will help to prevent water discolouration, tastes, odours and the proliferation of microorganisms (which may create a food-chain leading to the appearance of animals such as crustaceans). The potential health significance of microorganisms growing in piped supply systems is discussed in Chapter 1. The presence of large numbers of bacteria in the conveyed water may make it difficult to identify serious contamination from outside the pipework and reservoir structures. Finally, the proliferation of nonpathogenic organisms may make water unpalatable and encourage recipients to consume an alternative, and possibly less safe, source of water.

This chapter looks at how treatment can be optimized to control microbial growth, corrosion of pipe materials and the formation of deposits such as biofilms and sediments. It is not a general guide to water treatment.

2.2 MICROBIAL GROWTH FACTORS

Biological activity in a distribution system is normally most intense at the interface between the water and structural materials (in formations generally described as biofilms), and within deposits formed by particulate matter and corrosion.

The growth of biofilms depends on the nature of the material, the hydraulic conditions and the physical and chemical characteristics of the water (Camper et al., 2000). Colonisation occurs from the first contact between certain microorganisms (mainly bacteria) and a new material. It then evolves through the integration of various levels and species that can cohabit and exchange nutrients by reacting to external conditions.

When a microbial biofilm has formed, or a deposit containing organic matter has precipitated, it can serve as a food source for predators such as protozoa, which may themselves be consumed by higher animals such as *Asellus aquaticus* (see Chapter 6).

The factors controlling microbial growth and development in distribution systems are shown in Figure 2.1. Some of these are discussed below.

- **Temperature** — If nutrients are available, the microbial activity (as measured by HPC) increases significantly at water temperatures above 15°C, in the absence of a disinfectant residual.

- **pH** — Most microorganisms survive at the pH values normally found in drinking-water.
- **Oxygen** — Water supplies are normally well aerated, which reduces the risk of microbially-induced corrosion, denitrification, sulfide production and other consequences of anaerobic stagnation. However, oxygen may not penetrate to the bottom layers of biofilms, corrosion tubercles, and other pipe deposits and reservoir sediments where anaerobes such as sulfate-reducing bacteria may proliferate.
- **Nutrients** — Although some microorganisms can survive on mineral elements, they are of little significance in distribution networks. However, many microorganisms can proliferate if there is sufficient dissolved or particulate organic matter containing carbon, nitrogen or phosphorus.

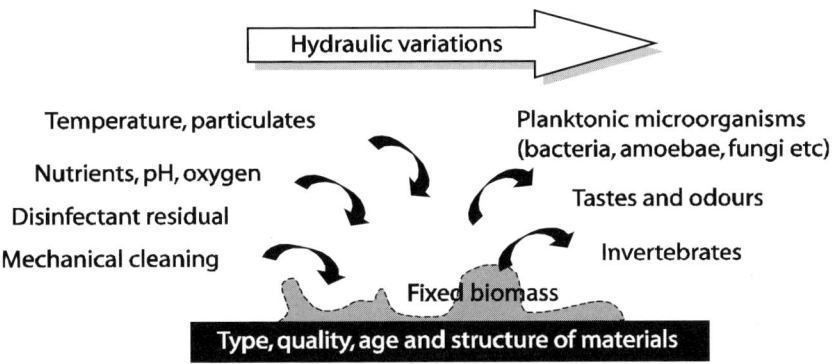

Figure 2.1. The factors influencing microbial change in water distribution systems.

2.3 TREATED WATER QUALITY OBJECTIVES

To prevent or minimize bacterial proliferation in distribution systems, the following general guidance should be followed:
- minimize particles leaving the treatment works;
- minimize the amount of particulate, colloidal and dissolved iron, manganese and aluminium compounds leaving the treatment works;
- restrict the biodegradable organic content leaving the works;
- control the corrosion potential of the water with respect to distribution system materials;
- minimize the factors causing the consumption of a residual disinfectant;
- adapt the disinfectant residual to the local conditions and climatic conditions;
- introduce a monitoring policy that can identify failures in achieving the above.

2.3.1 Disinfection strategy and the distribution system

The disinfectant concentration and contact time applied must be appropriate for the prevailing water temperature and pH, and for the target microorganisms. This is best achieved within a contact tank at the treatment plant where the hydraulics are designed to ensure effective contact between microorganisms and disinfectant. Details may be found in the companion volume addressing drinking-water treatment (LeChevallier et al., 2003). In some countries, transmission mains may be used for ensuring such contact. If so, it is important to ensure that there are no side connections or branches before full disinfection has been achieved under well-controlled contact conditions. In reality, this may be difficult to achieve.

Residual disinfectant will be consumed by corrosion products on the internal surface of metal piping, by iron and manganese deposits from corrosion and carry-over from the plant, by organic biomasses and by part of the organic matter circulating in the water. Therefore, maintenance of a residual is assisted by control of corrosion, treatment that minimizes carry-over of particulates and coagulant, low levels of dissolved organic matter, a system that is free of all types of deposit and short water-transmission times between the treatment plant and the consumer.

Chlorine, chloramines and chlorine dioxide are the three disinfectants that have been used to maintain a residual in distribution. Ozone decays too rapidly for this application. The selection of the most appropriate chemical and its dose depends on the microbial water quality targets or performance targets (see WHO, 2004). Selection also depends on the risks of developing tastes, odours and disinfection by-products such as trihalomethanes (THMs) at the point of disinfection and within the network. This decision can be complex. In many situations, the choice is also dependent on the performance of available dosing and monitoring equipment.

Chlorine

Chlorine is commonly used to maintain a residual. Its disinfecting power is a function of pH, because when chlorine is added to water it reacts to produce hypochlorous acid (HOCl):

$$Cl_2 + H_2O \rightarrow HOCl + H^+ + Cl^-$$

The hypochlorous acid will dissociate to the hypochlorite ion (OCl$^-$) as the water increases in pH:

$$HOCl \rightarrow H^+ + OCl^-$$

The hypochlorite ion is a less powerful disinfectant than hypochlorous acid. Table 2.1 shows how the proportion of the hypochlorite ion increases with pH.

Table 2.1. Dissociation of hypochlorous acid as a function of pH

pH	% HOCl	% OCl⁻
7	78	22
8	28	72
9	4	96
10	0	100

Source: Snoeyink & Jenkins (1980)

The correct selection and control of pH is therefore crucial for effective disinfection at the treatment works when using chlorine. This is less important when seeking to maintain a residual because the hypochlorite ion, although less effective, will decay more slowly and will thus persist further into the network for a particular dose. In Europe, common target concentrations for free chlorine residual at the tap are 0.1–0.3 mg/l. At the higher value, consumers commonly detect the taste and odour of chlorine. However, detection levels vary widely between people and some can detect chlorine at much lower levels. (Complaints generally occur in response to changes in concentration rather than to consistent values, whether high or low.) In some countries, much higher concentrations have been employed to maintain a residual (UKWIR, 1998a).

The formation of THMs must be considered when maintaining chlorine residual. Applying adequate treatment before distribution minimizes organic precursor compounds (Carlson, 1991) and is thus important in controlling THMs. If organic precursors to THMs remain, further chlorination may create THMs. The factors affecting the formation of THMs (UKWIR, 2000c) are:

- *pH* — about 10–20% more THMs will form at pH 9 than at pH 7;
- *time* — the rate of formation of THMs is greatest during the first 2–20 hours;
- *temperature* — at $< 10^{\circ}C$, THM concentrations do not increase significantly;
- *total organic carbon (TOC)* — at values of TOC above 4 mg/l it will be difficult to prevent THMs exceeding 100 µg/l if free chlorine is maintained to the tap for travel times of 2–3 days.

Monochloramine

A monochloramine residual may have advantages over a free chlorine residual (for a health-related benefit, see Box 2.1). In water, ammonia and chlorine react to form monochloramine (NH_2Cl), dichloramine ($NHCl_2$) and nitrogen trichloride (NCl_3). The chloramines are less powerful disinfectants than free chlorine, and are therefore often used as a secondary rather than a primary disinfectant within the treatment plant. However, they do persist in distribution (decay rates can be up to 20 times slower than free chlorine). Nitrogen trichloride produces a strong taste and odour at concentrations above 0.02 mg/l, whereas taste and odour thresholds for monochloramine are between 0.48 and 0.65 mg/l. High concentrations of dichloramine (> 0.15 mg/l) may produce tastes and odours. It is, therefore, important to control the disinfection process to produce a stable residual that is predominantly monochloramine. This requires evaluation of the water in question as a function of temperature, but normally a molar ratio of chlorine to ammonia of one and a pH value above seven is required (Snoeyink & Jenkins, 1980; Palin, 1975).

Monochloramine residuals in distribution will not increase THMs, although the process of chloramination can give rise to these chemicals, because free chlorine will be present at some point in the process. However, if this step is well managed it will be short lived, and any THMs formed will be at low concentrations. Monochloramine is more effective than free chlorine at penetrating and inactivating organisms within biofilms, especially where corrosion products are present (LeChevallier et al., 1993; Norton, 1995). Chloramination has also been found to be effective in controlling *Naegleria fowleri* in Australian water supplies (Christy & Robinson, 1984; UWRAA, 1990).

Treatment to produce a monochloramine residual does pose the risk of nitrite formation in the distribution system, especially in low-flow stagnant areas. Bacteria on surfaces and in deposits may nitrify any slight excess of ammonia. However, careful control of the chloramination process will prevent most nitrite problems (Williams, Andrews & Wakeford, 2001). If nitrite does occur at certain locations, despite good control of the chloramination process, then the presence of internal pipe deposits at these locations should be investigated.

Chlorine dioxide

Chlorine dioxide is a powerful biocide and is used in treatment works, especially where there is a problem with THM production. However, chlorine dioxide in water produces inorganic breakdown products, chlorite and chlorate. The health significance of chlorite and chlorate in drinking-water is discussed in the third edition of WHO *Guidelines for Drinking-water Quality* (WHO, 2004). The persistence of chlorine dioxide in distribution is unclear. Microbial aftergrowth in the presence of chlorine dioxide has occurred in some systems. This has been explained by rapid conversion of chlorine dioxide to chlorite in distribution systems and the subsequent measurement of chlorite rather than the dioxide (Brett & Ridgway, 1981). Therefore, any attempt to maintain a chlorine dioxide residual would require careful investigation.

> **Box 2.1.** Disinfection and the risk of legionnaires' disease.
>
> The authors conducted a retrospective case-control study to identify risk factors for hospital outbreaks of legionnaires' disease. They identified 32 hospitals where one or more outbreaks had been identified between 1979 and 1997. In addition, 48 control hospitals, matched for size and whether they had transplant programmes, were identified.
>
> Case-hospitals were far more likely to be supplied with water that contained free chlorine (rather than monochloramine) as a residual disinfectant than were control hospitals (adjusted odds ratio 10.2, 95% confidence intervals 1.4 to 460). The authors estimated that about 90% of all hospital outbreaks of legionnaires' disease could be prevented if all water utilities in the USA switched to chloramination.
>
> The suggestion is that monochloramine residual disinfection is more effective at inhibiting the growth of biofilm in water distribution systems, and that this in turn affects the risk of legionnaires' disease. This is an example of how disinfection practice can affect the quality and safety of water in distribution.
> Source: Kool, Carpenter & Fields (1999).

Management of disinfectant residuals

Not all countries have the same attitude to the maintenance of disinfectant residuals in distribution systems. Water suppliers in many European countries, for example, are seeking to reduce the use of chlorine and its derivatives wherever it is feasible to do so, by optimising treatment to remove organic material.

Hydraulics simulation models and results of microbiological analysis can be used to optimize the management of disinfectant residuals (Heraud et al., 1997; Dukan et al., 1996; Piriou et al., 1997). Controlling disinfectant residuals by booster dosing (re-dosing with a disinfectant at strategic points in the network) is described in Chapter 3. Modelling the concentration of a disinfectant in distribution requires knowledge of its reactivity with:

- the treated water (e.g. chlorine is consumed rapidly at first, followed by an on-going but slow process);
- the pipe deposits and biofilms present in the system;
- the pipeline and network construction materials (information on the chlorine and monochloramine demand of common distribution materials is available (UKWIR, 1998b; AWWARF, 1998)).

Such modelling requires specialist knowledge, but can assist in optimising the treatment process or identifying the network locations where booster disinfection will be most effective.

2.3.2 Particulate content, turbidity and coagulant residual

Particles capable of surviving the various phases of drinking-water treatment can transport microorganisms adsorbed on their surface, fixed as biofilm or integrated into the porous mass. They may be protected from an oxidizing disinfectant if the particles contain reducing compounds, such as iron oxides or organic matter. If ultraviolet (UV) light irradiation is used, the shadow cones projected by the particle mass can limit the effectiveness of this disinfecting procedure. Thus, achieving turbidities of less than 1.0 nephelometric turbidity unit (NTU) in waters entering distribution will significantly reduce the risk of breakthrough of pathogenic microorganisms, many of which may be resistant to disinfection.

The particles that settle in the network may eventually form adhesive deposits and sediments in reservoirs and pipes where microorganisms will be protected. This causes a secondary problem if changes in flow direction and velocity resuspend these deposits and associated microorganisms, contaminating the water supply.

Another common cause of particulate formation in distribution arises from the by-products of water treatment processes (e.g. where iron and aluminium compounds are used as flocculants). Water that complies with recommended metal concentrations on health and aesthetic grounds may contain sufficient material to precipitate as deposits in the distribution system (UKWIR, 2000a). Post-treatment deposition of iron and aluminium coagulant, manganese and silica has been observed (WRc, 1981). There is no generally applicable guidance for the residual concentrations of these components of treated water to avoid such deposition problems. It is therefore prudent to routinely monitor not only the composition of water leaving a treatment works but also the composition during passage to the extremities of the network to reveal deposition processes. In the United Kingdom, the recommendations shown in Table 2.2 have been made for water leaving treatment works.

Information is available on procedures for identifying and rectifying process conditions that lead to such problems, and for identifying where such post-treatment works precipitation is occurring (WRc, 1990).

Table 2.2. Recommended values for UK final waters to reduce deposition in distribution.

Determinand	Suggested maximum[a]	Suggested target[b]
Iron (mg/l)	0.10	0.05
Aluminium (mg/l)	0.10	0.05
Manganese (mg/l)	0.05	0.025
Turbidity (NTU)	0.50	1.00

NTU = nephelometric turbidity unit
Source: a, WRc (1990); b, UKWIR (2000a)

2.3.3 Organic matter

In recent years, attention has focused on the carbonaceous organic matter that can be used by microorganisms as a source of nutrients. Among the various parameters published by research teams, two have been made into international standards: biodegradable dissolved organic carbon (BDOC) and assimilable organic carbon (AOC). The purpose of these parameters is to measure the nutritional potential of water directly or indirectly in terms of carbonaceous organic compounds (Kaplan, Reasoner & Rice, 1994); they are not intended for routine monitoring. In the terminology of water safety plans, these parameters are used for "process validation" (see Section 7.3.3). They must be studied in depth during an investigational stage in order to understand fully how they develop in the source water and evolve throughout the treatment process. Thus, they serve to optimize the process and provide information during pilot testing, with a view to modifying or designing the treatment plant. The parameters will then be checked only periodically to verify the performance of the treatment works.

Assimilable organic carbon

This parameter was developed by Van der Kooij (1992). It is based on culturing two bacterial strains in the water under investigation and matching the maximum number of cells obtained with a calibration curve produced by using an easily assimilated nutrient such as sodium acetate (APHA-AWWA-WEF, 1995). After many years of experience, Van der Kooij has been able to establish an AOC scale that allows waters to be classified in terms of bacterial regrowth potential. A value of no more than 10 µg/l of AOC from the *Pseudomonas* p17 strain is recommended for biologically stable water. The AOC level is considered to indicate the quantity of carbon in a test water that can easily be assimilated by bacteria.

Biodegradable dissolved organic carbon

The sample to be analysed is placed in contact with a native mixed biomass. Monitoring of the dissolved organic carbon (DOC) enables the degradation of the organic matter to be observed, with the corresponding increase in carbon dioxide and bacterial cells (Figure 2.2). When the degradation has reached a plateau, the value obtained is described as refractory dissolved organic carbon (RDOC). The difference between the initial DOC and the RDOC enables the BDOC to be calculated in milligrams per litre (Block et al., 1992). A 30-day incubation method has been published (Servais, Anzil & Ventresque, 1989). For a faster result, Joret & Levi (1986) incubated the sample on a mass of colonised sand, generally taken from the sand filters of treatment plants. This sand contains a native biomass that is well adapted to the water under investigation and can completely degrade the BDOC in 5–7 days. These two methods have been compared by Volk et al. (1994).

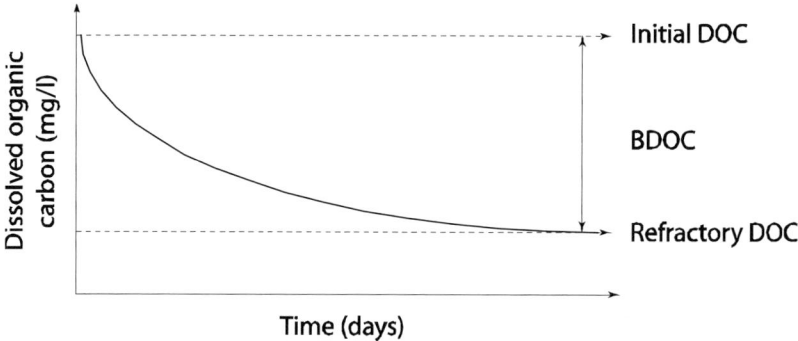

Figure 2.2. An example of a typical biodegradation curve for dissolved organic carbon (DOC).

The method allows quantification not only of the easily assimilable carbon but also of the carbon that will be degraded by bacteria more slowly during distribution. It has been found that waters that are biologically stable in distribution have BDOC values of 0.2 mg/l or less. Comparisons of the methods have shown that AOC is the most easily assimilated fraction of the BDOC. Whichever method is used, ozonation has been found to lead to conversion of refractory TOC into biodegradable TOC. Consequently, the use of ozone is not recommended during the final treatment stages before distribution (Joret, Levi & Volk, 1991; Volk & LeChevallier, 1999).

Biofilm formation potential

Methods for assessing biofilm formation potential combine information about the dissolved organic content with an evaluation of its potential to promote the proliferation of fixed biomasses.

One of these methods determines the biofilm formation potential (BFP) parameter (Van der Kooij & Veenendal, 1992). The water under investigation is percolated continuously through a device containing glass cylinders. At regular intervals, a cylinder is sampled and the fixed biomass estimated by calculating the metabolic activity. This is achieved by measuring the level of adenosine triphosphate (ATP, a component of all living microbial cells) using luminescence. Plotting the kinetics allows different waters to be compared, and investigators in the Netherlands have used this technique to identify water resources that are more likely to support biofilm formation in distribution systems (Van den Hoven et al., 1996).

A European task force has worked on the development of a similar method that is simple, easy and cheap, and does not require complex equipment (AGHTM, 1999). The water is percolated through a bed of glass beads and the biomass is assessed by bacterial counts on R2A agar or by measuring ATP, total protein or TOC. The protocol has been validated but results vary between laboratories.

Although these methods are not the subject of international standardization, they can be used to select water resources and treatment options for minimizing biodegradable organic matter entering distribution systems. However, due to difficulties with interlaboratory comparability, the analysis must be done systematically by the same individuals using the same methods, to limit the variability of results.

2.3.4 Limiting the potential for corrosion and scale

Internal corrosion of iron pipes reduces their structural strength and may create leaks and bursts, as does external corrosion. Internal corrosion also increases the consumption of disinfectant residual, decreases the water-carrying capacity of the pipe and creates deposits that are undesirable in terms of maintaining high microbial quality (LeChevallier et al., 1993). The internal corrosion of the traditional cast and ductile iron pipes, protected by a paint layer of coal-tar (no longer recommended due to leaching of polycyclic aromatic hydrocarbons), often produces hard adhesive tubercles, as shown in Plate 2.1.

In unprotected steel pipes, the corrosion products tend to be more uniform and less adhesive. Other scales based on adhesive and layered calcium carbonate deposits can form in mains when the conveyed water is excessively supersaturated with calcium carbonate. These may also be found in association with corrosion products and biofilms (Lu, Kiene & Levi, 1998). Calcium carbonate deposits and ferrous corrosion products usually require mechanical action or an acid chemical process for their removal.

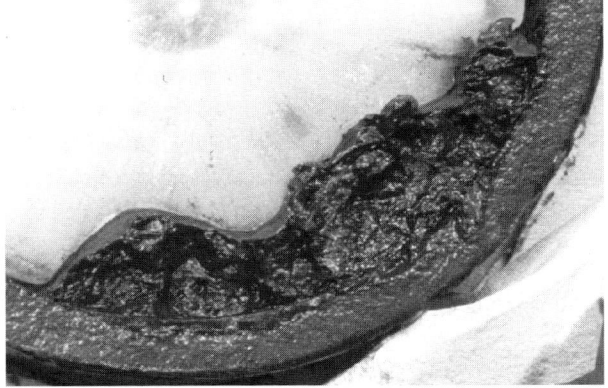

Plate 2.1. Corrosion tubercles in 40 year old cast iron main (100 mm diameter).

To prevent corrosion and scale, the water should be saturated or slightly over-saturated with calcium carbonate (Legrand & Leroy, 1995).

Several options are available for controlling the corrosivity of treated water towards the range of materials used in the distribution network. These should be considered on a case-by-case basis. It is also important to consider how changes in water composition may affect the corrosion of all distribution and plumbing materials. Guidance is available for minimizing corrosion in networks containing pipes made from iron, lead, copper, galvanised steel and cement-based materials (UKWIR, 2000b).

2.4 OPTIMIZATION OF TREATMENT

2.4.1 Water sources

Where there is a choice of water source, content of biodegradable organic matter should be considered. Protected underground resources or sites, where there can be groundwater replenishment or bank infiltration, are preferred. In most circumstances, the quality of groundwater improves during its passage through subterranean rocks and subsoils, resulting in more biologically stable water entering the distribution system. In contrast, surface waters containing a lot of humus-based material, urban or industrial effluents, or a proliferation of algae are more difficult to treat and are more likely to contain a high proportion of undesirable nutrients.

For small, community-managed systems, the selection of source waters with lower potential for promoting regrowth is preferred, given the usually limited availability of water-quality testing equipment and lack of skills in interpreting the results of microbiological analysis. However, the overriding requirement should still be the selection of sources with the lowest risk of contamination with pathogens.

2.4.2 Drinking-water treatment plant

The water treatment plant should be designed and operated to minimize dissolved and particulate nutrient entering the network. The processes include biodegradation, retention and adsorption (Jacangelo et al., 1995), summarized below.

A preliminary stage of biological nitrification will remove ammonia without using chlorine, thus limiting the formation of unwanted by-products. However, the biodegradation will not be effective below 5°C, and if nitrification stops during prolonged periods of low temperatures, it will be necessary to use a stand-by chemical method.

Flocculation must be optimized by selecting the best flocculant and the best pH, not just to reduce turbidity but also to reduce both colloidal and dissolved organic matter. If this stage is well managed, it can also reduce some undesirable organic micropollutants and disinfection by-product precursors (Crozes, White & Marshall, 1995). The chemistry of the coagulation process must also be controlled to minimize carry-over of dissolved and colloidal coagulant. This is especially important in waters of low calcium hardness (WRc, 1992).

Some clarifiers, like the floc blanket reactors that promote prolonged contact between the water and the microorganisms held in the sludge, allow a biodegradation stage to be introduced at the beginning of the treatment cycle (Campos et al., 1999a). The addition of powdered activated carbon may be used to reduce the DOC content.

Biological sand filters have a biodegrading effect because of the biomass that develops in the first few tens of centimetres. The particle size and contact time must promote good contact between the organic carbon and the biomass. Generally, the bacteria must not come into contact with disinfectants used during water pretreatment or in the filter cleaning water, because this would slow down the biological activity in the filters (Laurent et al., 1999a). Monitoring is essential to identify any risk of excessive growth, which could cause blockages in the filter mass and thereby limit the effectiveness of filter backwashing (Croue et al., 1997). Rapid filtration usually results in a BDOC reduction of 20–30%, as long as the water does not contain disinfectant residual.

Dune, riverbank and soil filtration are very effective methods if the residence times are long enough. In addition to the removal of particulate matter and microorganisms, BDOC may be considerably reduced, ensuring stability in the distribution system.

The biocidal and oxidizing effects of ozonation can be highly beneficial. However, ozonation converts refractory organic matter into biodegradable organic matter (Ribas et al., 1997). This effect can neutralize the BDOC improvement produced by a preliminary sand filtration stage, creating a need for further biological filtration downstream (Van der Kooij, Hijnen & Kruithof, 1989; Volk et al., 1993).

Filtration through granular activated carbon (GAC) in the adsorption mode can reduce organic carbon in a controlled way. However, the GAC will become saturated with organic compounds quite quickly, which means that frequent regeneration will be required, according to the type of water. The presence of an active microbial biomass can slow the saturation of the GAC due to breakdown of the adsorbed organic materials. The choice of the type and brand of carbon must be based on a preliminary pilot study over several months on-site, to observe the adsorption decline pattern and the progressive emergence of the degrading biomass. The process cannot be simulated in the laboratory or by short-term experiments (Bablon, Ventresque & Benaïm, 1988). Low temperatures do not favour the generation of active biomass.

Recent studies have shown that the combined use of powdered carbon and ultrafiltration can eliminate not only the finest particles, bacteria and protozoa, but also a large proportion of the TOC (Clark, Baudin & Anselme, 1996; Campos et al., 1999b).

Membrane retention of TOC will also remove a large proportion of mineral salts, without the use of activated carbon. Some form of remineralisation or treatment with corrosion inhibitor may then be required to prevent corrosion in the distribution system (Agbekodo, Legube & Cote, 1996; Laurent et al., 1999b).

Box 2.2. Water quality deterioration associated with a change in disinfection practice.

In the late summer of 2000, the water supply in the City of Coquitlam, Canada, had high total coliform counts, though indicators of faecal contamination had been negative.

The supply came from surface water in mountainous areas and was treated by newly introduced coarse screening and chlorination. In May 2000, an ozone treatment facility had been commissioned to treat water before chlorination and distribution. With the onset of ozonation there was an increase in assimilable organic carbon (AOC) and biodegradable dissolved organic carbon (BDOC) in water entering the distribution system.

The supply area varied in elevation from 64 to 390 m. Water for consumers at the highest point travelled through a series of service reservoirs until it reached the highest storage tank (summit), some 420 m above sea level. Chlorine levels declined through each reservoir, from 0.7 to 0.8 mg/l at the treatment works to about 0.4 mg/l in the lowest reservoir, and less than 0.05 mg/l at the summit. In the autumn of 2000, there had been several high total coliform counts in the area of distribution served by the two highest reservoirs. High heterotrophic plate counts were common in these parts of the system as well. The positive total coliform counts led to the issue of advice to boil drinking-water.

The cause of this coliform bloom was a combination of the increase in AOC and BDOC (produced by ozonation), combined with low chlorine levels in the distal part of the system. The two highest reservoirs had particularly large storage in relation to demand, with the summit reservoir holding almost seven days supply and the next highest four days. The problem was resolved by regular cleaning of reservoirs and flushing of mains, reducing residence times in the service reservoirs and installing additional chlorination equipment.

Although coliform blooms as reported here do not represent a risk to human health, advice to boil water was issued. Boil water advice may carry its own risks to public health from scalds, anxiety and increased costs.

Source: Gehlen et al. (2002)

2.4.3 Decentralized treatment

The development of larger urban areas and the difficulties of building large treatment works in cities leads to more extensive distribution systems. In these situations, it may be necessary to adjust water quality in the distribution network. For example, recent investigations have demonstrated the feasibility of using membrane technology for treating water in an urban distribution network (Levi et al., 1997).

Chlorination booster stations (also known as relay stations) are commonly used in networks to manage chlorine residuals. They avoid the need for excessively high doses of disinfectant at treatment works to ensure that residuals reach the extremities of a network. The locations of rechlorination stations can be optimized using hydraulic models to simulate the residence times and the disinfectant residual (see Chapter 3). The effects of water temperature should be included, to avoid overdosing and prevent excessive formation of by-products in certain seasons of the year. However, booster chlorination should not be regarded as a means of preventing contamination of the distribution system (Snead et al., 1980) or as an alternative to monitoring system performance.

2.5 SUMMARY

It is not meaningful or practicable to strive for a sterile drinking-water network devoid of all microorganisms. Although the presence of nonpathogenic organisms does not directly threaten public health, their proliferation may make water unpalatable and encourage recipients to consume an alternative, and possibly less safe, source of water. In addition, the presence of large numbers of bacteria in the conveyed water, or in biofilms and deposits, may compromise the identification of serious contamination from outside the pipework and reservoir structures.

The optimization of treatment to minimize the amount of microbial nutrients and deposit-forming components entering the network will help to prevent water discolouration, tastes, odours and the proliferation of microorganisms. Optimization of treatment should be the first stage in any plan to ensure the microbial quality of water during distribution. Once deposits and biofilms have formed in a system, they are difficult to remove.

Water treatment can be optimized to prevent microbial growth, corrosion of pipe materials and the formation of deposits by adopting the following practices:
- continuous and reliable elimination of particles and the production of water of low turbidity;
- precipitation and removal of dissolved (and particulate) iron and manganese;

- minimization of the carry-over of residual coagulant (either dissolved, colloidal or particulate) that may precipitate in reservoirs and pipework;
- reduction (as far as possible) of dissolved organic matter, especially AOC and BDOC, that provides carbon-based nutrients for microorganisms;
- maintenance of the corrosion potential within limits that avoid damage to the structural materials and consumption of disinfectant;
- production of water with a low disinfectant demand, enabling disinfectant residuals to be maintained throughout the network without giving rise to unwanted by-products;
- adaptation of the disinfectant residual and its control to local conditions and climatic variation.

Predicting the effects of treatment options to minimize biological degradation in the network is not readily achieved using laboratory simulations. However, measurements of operationally-defined parameters such as AOC or BDOC can be used to evaluate the relative effects of different treatment processes designed to remove organic nutrients.

2.6 REFERENCES

AWWARF (1998). *Development of disinfection guidelines for the installation and replacement of water mains.* American Water Works Association Research Foundation, Denver, USA, 55.

Agbekodo KM, Legube B, Cote P (1996). Nanofiltration yields high quality drinking water in Paris suburb. *Journal of the American Water Works Association*, 88:67–74

AGHTM Biofilm Group (1999) Standard method to evaluate aquatic biofilms. In: Keevil CW, ed. *Biofilm in the aquatic environment.* Royal Society of Chemistry, 210–219.

APHA–AWWA–WEF (1995) *Standard methods for the examination of water and wastewater*, 19th ed. American Public Health Association, Washington DC.

Armon R et al. (1997). Survival of *Legionella pneumophila* and *Salmonella typhimurium* in biofilm systems. *Water Science and Technology*, 35(11–12):293–300.

Bablon GP, Ventresque C, Benaïm R (1988). Developing a sand GAC filter to achieve high rate biological filtration. *Journal of the American Water Works Association*, 80:47–53.

Block JC et al. (1992). Indigenous bacterial inocula for measuring the biodegradable dissolved organic carbon in waters. *Water Research*, 26:481–486

Brett RW, Ridgway JW (1981). Experiences with chlorine dioxide in Southern Water Authority and Water Research Centre. *Journal of the Institution of Water Engineers and Scientists*, 35:135–142.

Camper AK et al. (2000). *Investigation of the biological stability of water in treatment plants and distribution systems.* American Water Works Association Research Foundation.

Campos C et al. (1999a). Application of powdered activated carbon to floc blanket reactors for the removal of trace organic compounds. *Proceedings of the American Water Works Association Annual Conference*, Chicago.

Campos C et al. (1999b). Effect of process design and operating procedures on the performance of PAC/UF systems for the removal of organic compounds. *Proceedings of the AWWA Membrane Technology Conference*, Long Beach, California.

Carlson M (1991). Disinfection by-products precursor removal. *Proceedings of the 1991 AWWA Annual Conference — Water research for the new decade*, 151–191.

Christy P and Robinson B (1984). Disinfection of water for control of amoebae. *Water* 11, 21–24.

Clark MM, Baudin I, Anselme C (1996). Membrane powdered activated carbon reactors. In: *Water treatment membrane processes*, McGraw-Hill, 15-1–15-22.

Croue JP et al. (1997). Impact des traitements de potabilisation sur le CODB et la distribution des substances humiques et non humiques de la matière organique naturelle. *Revue des Sciences de l'Eau*, 1:63–81.

Crozes G, White P, Marshal M (1995). Enhanced coagulation: its effect on NOM removal and chemical costs. *Journal of the American Water Works Association*, 87(1):78–89

Dukan S et al. (1996) Dynamic modelling of bacterial growth in drinking water networks. *Water Research*, 30(9):1991–2002.

Gehlen IJ et al. (2002). Addressing heterotrophic bacteria regrowth in the city of Coquitlam water distribution system. In: *Proceedings of the NSF International / World Health Organization Symposium on HPC Bacteria in Drinking water*, April 22–24, 2002, Geneva, Switzerland, 479–500.

Heraud J et al. (1997). Optimised modelling of chlorine residual in a drinking water distribution system with a combination of on-line sensors. *Journal of Water Supply: Research and Technology — Aqua*, 46:1–12.

Jacangelo JG et al. (1995). Selected processes for removing NOM : an overview. *Journal of the American Water Works Association*, 87:64–77.

Joret JC, Levi Y (1986). Méthode rapide d'évaluation du carbone éliminable des eaux par voie biologique. *Tribune du Cebedeau*, 510(39):3–9.

Joret JC, Levi Y, Volk C (1991). Biodegradable dissolved organic carbon (BDOC) content of drinking water and potential regrowth of bacteria. *Water Science and Technology*, 24(2):95–101.

Kaplan LA, Reasoner DJ, Rice EW (1994). A survey of BOM in US drinking waters. *Journal of the American Water Works Association*, 86:121–132.

Kool JL, Carpenter JC, Fields BS (1999). Effect of monochloramine disinfection of municipal drinking water on risk of nosocomial Legionnaires' disease. *Lancet*, 353:272–77.

Laurent P et al. (1999a) Biodegradable organic matter removal in biological filters: evaluation of the chabrol model. *Water Research*, 33(6):1387–1398.

Laurent P et al. (1999b). Microbiological quality before and after nanofiltration. *Journal of the American Water Works Association*, 91(10)62–72.

LeChevallier MW et al. (1993) Examining the relationship between iron corrosion and the disinfection of biofilm bacteria. *Journal of the American Water Works Association*, 85:111–123.

LeChevallier MW et al. (2003). *Drinking-water treatment and water quality: the impact of treatment on microbial water quality and occurrence of pathogens and indicators in surface water.* WHO, Geneva and IWA Publishing, London.

Legrand L, Leroy P (1995). *Prevention de la corrosion et de l'entartrage dans les réseaux de distribution d'eau.* Ed. CIFEC, France.

Levi Y et al. (1997). Demonstration unit of satellite treatment in distribution system using ultrafiltration and nanofiltration. *Proceedings of the American Water Works Association Membrane Technology Conference*, New Orleans, 1997, 581–595.

Lu W, Kiene L, Levi Y (1998). Chlorine demand of biofilms in water distribution systems. *Water Research*, 33(3):827–835.

Norton CD (1995). *Implementation of chloramination and corrosion control to limit microbial activity in the distribution system.* American Water Works Service Company Report.

Palin AT (1975). Water disinfection — chemical aspects and analytical control. In: Johnson JD, ed. *Disinfection — water and wastewater*. Ann Arbor Science, Ann Arbor, Michigan, USA.

Piriou P et al. (1997). Prevention of bacterial growth in drinking water distribution systems. *Water Science and Technology*, 35(11–12):283–287.

Ribas F et al. (1997). Efficiency of various water treatment processes in the removal of biodegradable and refractory organic matter. *Water Research*, 31(3):639-649.

Servais P, Anzil A, Ventresque C (1989). Simple method for the determination of biodegradable dissolved organic carbon in water. *Applied and Environmental Microbiology*, 55(10):2732–2734.

Snead MC et al. (1980) The effectiveness of chlorine residuals in inactivation of bacteria and viruses introduced by post-treatment contamination. *Water Research*, 14:403–408.

Snoeyink VL, Jenkins D (1980). *Water chemistry*. Wiley, New York.

UKWIR (1998a). *Impact of service pipes on the bacteriological quality of water supplies*. Report 98/DW/02/15, UK Water Industry Research Limited, London.

UKWIR (1998b). *Chlorine and monochloramine demand of materials*. Report 98/DW/03/9, UK Water Industry Research Limited, London.

UKWIR (2000a). *Toolboxes for maintaining and improving drinking water quality*. Report 00/DW/03/11, Section 4, Toolbox for Iron Discolouration and Particulates, UK Water Industry Research Limited, London.

UKWIR (2000b). *Toolboxes for maintaining and improving drinking water quality*. Report 00/DW/03/11, Section 8, Toolbox for pH, UK Water Industry Research Limited, London.

UKWIR (2000c). *Toolboxes for maintaining and improving drinking water quality*. Report 00/DW/03/11, Section 3, Toolbox for Trihalomethane Formation, UK Water Industry Research Limited, London.

UWRAA (Urban Water Research Association of Australia) (1990) Report No 15 Chloramination of Water Supplies. Water Services Association of Australia.

Van den Hoven T et al. (1996). Simplified methods to monitor water quality changes in distribution systems. *Water Supply*, 14(3/4):515–533.

Van der Kooij D, Hijnen WAM, Kruithof JC (1989). The effects of ozonation, biological filtration and distribution on the concentration of easily assimilable organic carbon (AOC) in drinking water. *Ozone: Science and Engineering*, 11:297–311.

Van der Kooij D (1992). Assimilable organic carbon as an indicator of bacterial regrowth. *Journal of the American Water Works Association*, 84:57–65.

Van der Kooij D, Veenendaal HR (1992). Assessment of the biofilm formation characteristics of drinking water. *Proceedings of the American Water Works Association Water Quality Technology Conference*, Toronto.

Volk C et al. (1993). Effects of ozone on the production of biodegradable dissolved organic carbon during water treatment. *Ozone: Science and Engineering*, 15:389–404.

Volk C et al. (1994). Comparison of two techniques for measuring biodegradable dissolved organic carbon in water. *Environmental Technology*, 15:546–556.

Volk C, LeChevallier MW (1999). Impacts of the reduction of nutrient levels on bacterial water quality in distribution systems. *Applied and Environmental Microbiology*, 65(11):4957–4966.

WHO (2004) *Guidelines for drinking-water quality*, 3rd ed. World Health Organization, Geneva.

Williams AM, Andrews S, Wakeford P (2001). The control of nitrite formation in London's distribution system. *Journal of the Chartered Institution of Water and Environmental Management*, 15:162–166.

WRc (1981). *A guide to solving water quality problems in distribution systems.* Technical Report TR167, Water Research Centre, Swindon, UK, 31.

WRc (1990). *Aesthetic water quality problems in distribution systems. A source document for the water mains rehabilitation manual.* Water Research Centre, Swindon, UK, 115.

WRc (1992). *Coagulant residuals in soft water.* Report no. 1330 UM, Water Research Centre, Swindon, UK.

3
Design and operation of distribution networks

Kay Chambers, John Creasey and Leith Forbes

3.1 INTRODUCTION

Water distribution networks serve many purposes in addition to the provision of water for human consumption, which often accounts for less than 2% of the total volume supplied. Piped water is used for washing, sanitation, irrigation and fire fighting. Networks are designed to meet peak demands; in parts of the network this creates low-flow conditions that can contribute to the deterioration of microbial and chemical water quality. To maintain microbial quality, the network should be designed and operated to prevent ingress of contaminants, to maintain disinfectant residual concentrations within a locally predetermined range and to minimize the transit time (or age of the water after leaving the treatment works).

© 2004 World Health Organization. *Safe Piped Water: Managing Microbial Water Quality in Piped Distribution Systems*. Edited by Richard Ainsworth. ISBN: 1 84339 039 6. Published by IWA Publishing, London, UK.

The issues for designing and operating a distribution network discussed in this chapter are:
- design and operation of piped networks;
- design and operation of service reservoirs;
- controlling disinfectant residuals by booster (relay) dosing;
- avoiding potential problems when mixing water sources in distribution;
- potential effects of zoning networks;
- pipe materials;
- pipe location;
- protection from cross-connections and backflow at point of delivery.

3.2 DESIGN AND OPERATION OF PIPED NETWORKS

3.2.1 Hydraulics

The purpose of a system of pipes is to supply water at adequate pressure and flow. However, pressure is lost by the action of friction at the pipe wall. The pressure loss is also dependent on the water demand, pipe length, gradient and diameter. Several established empirical equations describe the pressure–flow relationship (Webber, 1971), and these have been incorporated into network modelling software packages to facilitate their solution and use.

When designing a piped system, the aim is to ensure that there is sufficient pressure at the point of supply to provide an adequate flow to the consumer. For example, in England and Wales, water companies are required to supply water to a single property at a minimum of 10 m head of pressure at the boundary stoptap with a flow rate of 9 l/min (OFWAT, 1999). This minimum pressure increases as the number of properties supplied through a single service pipe increases.

For the purposes of maintaining microbial quality, it is important to minimize transit times and avoid low flows and pressures. These requirements have to be balanced against the practicalities of supplying water according to the location of consumers and where pipes can be laid.

Excessive capacity

The system should not have excessive capacity (which will result in long transit times) unless this excess capacity is required to meet a known increase in future demand.

Low-flow dead-ends and loops

Ideally, low-flow dead-ends and loops should be avoided, but in practice this is not always possible. Low-flow sections of dead-ends should be as short as possible. Both dead-ends and loops in the system may cause problems by creating long residence times and sections where sediments can collect. Changes in flow direction ("tidal flows") in loops may disturb any deposits in the pipes. Operators should be aware of these possible problematic locations and closely monitor and maintain these pipes (see Chapter 4).

Negative pressures

Situations that may give rise to negative pressures should always be avoided. Faecal organisms and culturable human viruses may be present in groundwater adjacent to a pipeline and drawn into a pipe during transient low or negative pressures (LeChevallier et al., 2003). Hydraulic models can be used to identify where, when and how negative pressures may occur. Preventative measures such as system reinforcement may then be identified and implemented. Until such measures are effective, staff responsible for the daily operation of the network should be informed of these situations and hence where, when and how contamination of the network may occur. Such situations may occur where there are:

- properties on high ground;
- remote properties at the end of long lengths of pipe;
- demands that are greater than the design demand;
- pipes of inadequate capacity (too small diameter);
- rough pipes (e.g. corroding iron pipes or pipes with a build-up of sediment);
- equipment failures (e.g. pumps and valves, see Section 3.2.2).

Appropriate pressures

Pressure at any point in the system should be maintained within a range whereby the maximum pressure avoids pipe bursts and the minimum ensures that water is supplied at adequate flow rates for all expected demands. This may require pressure boosting at strategic locations in the network (see Section 3.2.2).

Hydraulic models

If available, network models of the system should be used to check that the system will be or is operating to the required standard. Models are valuable during design and operation of a system. A model can be used to identify problems in an existing system (e.g. closed valves that should be open) by comparing modelled pressures with actual pressures in the system.

> **Box 3.1.** A hepatitis outbreak affecting a football team.
>
> During September and October 1969, hepatitis affected members of a football team at a college in Massachusetts, USA. Of 97 potentially exposed individuals, there was biochemical evidence that 90 were infected, of whom 32 were jaundiced, 22 were ill though not jaundiced and 36 had no symptoms. The clustering of cases suggested a common source. No cases were seen in other students on campus and the only common factor in affected individuals was attendance at the training ground. In the absence of alternative explanations, attention turned towards a possible water source at the training grounds.
>
> The water supply to the training ground was from a municipal supply and was used for both irrigation and drinking. The training ground was at the highest point on campus, about 80 m above the lowest point. The municipal system terminated at a meter pit and from there a pipe passed along the side of two fields, terminating at a hut where the drinking-water tap was situated. Subsurface taps used to irrigate the field were located at several points along the pipe.
>
> The water pressure in the municipal supply averaged 140 pounds per square inch (psi), though at peak demand the pressure was only 40 psi. It was noted that the pressure in the water pipe at the field was very variable and became negative when a couple of fire hydrants in the municipal supply were opened.
>
> Further investigations found that children who lived next to the practice field had suffered infectious hepatitis four weeks earlier and that these children played in the water that collected around one of the subsurface irrigation taps. Furthermore, at about the time that the cases would have been infected there had been a fire two miles away from the training grounds, along the line of the municipal supply. The conclusion was that the water around the irrigation tap had become contaminated from the children, that water demand from the fire had led to negative pressure in the field supply and that this had drawn contaminated water into the pipework.
>
> Source: Morse et al. (1972).

Intermittent supply

In some situations, water supplies are only available for a restricted number of hours per day or days per week. Although such systems are not desirable, they are the reality for a large proportion of the world's population. The control of water quality in intermittent supplies represents a significant challenge to water suppliers, because the risk of backflow increases significantly due to reduced pressure. The risk may be elevated in seasons with greater rainfall, where soil moisture conditions will increase the likelihood of a pressure gradient developing from the soil to the pipe. Within the supply, the most significant points of risk will be areas where pipes pass through drains or other places where stagnant water pools may form. Water quality may also deteriorate on recharging where surges may dislodge biofilm, leading to aesthetic problems.

Intermittent systems are very common in many countries; therefore, it is important to minimize the associated health risks. As discussed in Chapter 7, understanding the system — its vulnerability and hazards that affect it — is crucial to the control of water quality. It is unlikely to be feasible to run the first charge of water to waste throughout the system, but this may be possible in selected areas of elevated risk (determined by the potential for contamination of the supply and the level of service). Control of hazards in the immediate vicinity of pipes is more important because intermittent systems are inherently vulnerable. In the longer term, the reduction of intermittence is important; in some areas this may actually be relatively easy to achieve by using or rehabilitating service reservoirs.

3.2.2 Pumps and control valves

If gravity is insufficient to supply water at an adequate pressure, then pumps need to be installed to boost the pressure. Pumps can be either permanently operational or intermittent. They can be controlled by a time-switch, pressure or a water level in a tank or reservoir. A back-up system (e.g. a standby pump) may be needed.

Control valves (e.g. pressure reducing valves, nonreturn valves and throttled valves) are designed to optimize the operation of a network with respect to pressure, water supply and energy costs. Some control valves can be controlled from a remote site. For example, a pressure-reducing valve can be controlled by the pressure at a site further downstream that is known to be the critical low-pressure point in the network. All of these control valves need to be designed correctly for their application. Regular maintenance (see Chapter 4) is a key to ensuring that water quality is not compromised. If pumps or valves fail, low or negative pressures can arise, and this can lead to ingress of contaminants into the system. The correct location and size of a pump or valve can be identified using a network-modelling software package (see Section 3.2.1). Pumps and valves should be operated to minimize surge effects (see Section 3.2.4). Other issues to be aware of are as follows.

- Double acting air valves and ball-type hydrants, which allow the ingress of air at low pressures, provide an opportunity for ingress of contaminants if the valve is submerged in its chamber. It is important to keep the chamber dry and free of debris.
- It is worthwhile installing washout valves in dead-ends to make water disposal more convenient (see Section 3.2.1).
- Nonreturn valves may be a sensible precaution on the supply inlet to premises where high back-pressures could be accidentally generated

(see Section 3.9). Potential hazards include industrial, commercial and agricultural premises, and major "domestic" institutions such as hospitals and university halls of residence that may have significant storage and internal distribution.

3.2.3 Access for maintenance

When designing a network, it is important to incorporate fixtures that can be maintained with minimal disruption to normal flow regimes, using hygienic operating and maintenance practices (see Chapter 4 for details of maintenance procedures). The following are examples of appropriate fixtures.

- Hydrants either side of a closed valve. Stagnant, dirty water can collect at dead-ends formed by closed valves. When the valve is operated, this water and any deposits can be conveyed into the network and to consumers. By flushing the hydrants, some or all of this water can be removed before operating the valve.
- By-passes for devices such as flow meters and pressure-reducing valves that allow the devices to be taken out of service for maintenance. It may also be appropriate to install a second device, so that there is always one in use while the other is maintained.
- Valve chambers that are large enough to allow maintenance and replacement and are well drained, to reduce the possibility of contaminant ingress.
- Sufficient valves to allow containment of a problem to small areas of the system. This means that pipework does not have to be completely drained in the event of a pipe break and that small parts of the network can be isolated when undertaking system modifications.
- Entry and exit points for mains cleaning.
- Disinfection injection points at critical points, for emergency disinfectant injection to maintain a disinfectant residual.

The location and depth of installation of pipelines are important, especially when sewerage systems are adjacent (see Section 3.8). In the event of a burst water pipe, the soil structure will be undermined. If a sewer is nearby there is a risk of raw sewage entering the pipe, especially if the pipe is at the same depth or lower than the sewer.

It is worth noting that trunk mains (usually ≥ 200 mm in diameter) are generally less easy to maintain than other pipes. This is because they usually have few, if any, access points and, if they are taken out of service for maintenance, then large numbers of consumers are affected. Operators need to be aware of the risks and issues associated with trunk mains in order to plan work.

3.2.4 Surge events

A surge in pressure and flow can occur when pumps are switched or when valves and hydrants are operated. Any change in flow can result in surge (e.g. pressure reducing valve hunting can cause a surge); however, the common causes are the operation of pumps, valves and hydrants. This can result in a deterioration of water quality because the surge can disturb deposits in the pipe or on the pipe wall. These operations may also cause low pressures that could allow ingress of contaminants. The risk of significant surge, and hence water quality problems, is greater in long unbranched pipes than in branched pipes, because branched pipes reduce surge.

Recommended techniques for avoiding surge effects

There are several techniques to avoid surge effects, three of which are described here.
- Place air vessels close to pumps and major valves. Air vessels are devices that have air trapped above the water. The water level changes as the pressure varies, dampening the surge event. The advantage of this system is that no power supply is needed, but the volume of air must be maintained (Wylie & Streeter, 1978).
- Control the rate of switching pumps to make the change in flow gradual, so that the network can absorb the effect of the change in flow (Wylie & Streeter, 1978).
- Operate valves and hydrants slowly. The reasoning behind this technique is the same as for control of pump switching.

As for all devices in a network, the devices associated with the above techniques need to be sized and maintained correctly. A pump at the exit of a treatment works or service reservoir (a source pump) requires an air vessel (if this is the chosen solution) to be located immediately downstream of the pump's nonreturn valve. For a pump within the network, the upstream and downstream sides may need to be protected; thus, the correctly sized air vessel would need to be placed upstream of the pump's nonreturn valve. For a valve where suppression is needed, two air vessels may be required, one either side of the valve, to protect the network.

Other events such as fire fighting, bursts and sudden increases in demand can cause surges. Air vessels can be used to counter these surge events by placing them at a range of sites, but costs and practicalities may limit their use.

Specialized software packages are available to determine the correct position and size of an air vessel, the rate of switching of a pump and rate of operations of a valve or hydrant. This is the only way to accurately plan antisurge techniques. Basic charts have been produced but these are inadequate for networks. Wylie & Streeter (1978) give a full description of the mechanisms and analysis of surge events.

It is possible to determine an approximate minimum safe value for the time to take to switch a pump or operate a valve (WRc, 2000). The time 't' (in seconds) should be greater than 2L/a, where 'L' (in metres) is the "characteristic" length of the network and 'a' is the wavespeed for the pipes (in metres per second). The characteristic length of the network in its simplest form is the length of pipe downstream of the source of the surge. In a complex network, it may be the sum of the pipe lengths. The constant 'a' depends on the pipe material and other factors. As a guide, 'a' equals 300–500 m/s for a plastic pipe, 1000–1300 m/s for an iron pipe and 900–1200 m/s for asbestos cement. The critical stage of moving a valve is when it is nearly closed. This is when the movement must be carried out slowly and the time 't' applies to this part of the movement.

Inadvisable techniques for avoiding surge effects

The following three methods have also been employed to relieve surge but are not recommended because the risk of ingress and contamination is too great and/or they are impractical:
- Pressure relief valves. These release water to the atmosphere to reduce pressure but cannot solve a low-pressure surge problem.
- Double acting air valves. These are the opposite of pressure relief valves, letting air into the network when the pressure drops. These valves limit low pressures but cannot alleviate high pressures.
- Surge shafts. These are towers open to the atmosphere, which are usually very tall in order to hold water to a height equivalent to the maximum pressure head. They act like air vessels.

3.2.5 Integrated operations

The operation of a network should not just be a collection of uncoordinated activities such as valve and pump operation (and maintenance activities — see Chapter 4) but should take account of the interactions between these activities. This requires an overall strategy adapted to local circumstances and applicable to all water quality issues, not just microbial quality. The activities that can be included in a strategy are numerous and may include those listed below (UKWIR, 2000a).
- Risk assessment of each activity (e.g. valve operation) before it is undertaken and identification of actions to minimize risk (see chapters 4, 5 and 7 for tools that could be used for assessments).
- Procedures for mains cleaning, mains laying, repairs and renovations (see chapters 4 and 5 for microbiological aspects of these).

- Coordination with fire fighting services on hydrant use and awareness of which areas may be at risk of loss of pressure.
- Procedures for operating valves, hydrant and other fixtures (see sections 3.2.3 and 3.2.4 on access for maintenance and prevention of surge events). Consider labelling fixtures as to their type, status and allowed operations.
- Service reservoir design, operation and maintenance requirements (see Section 3.3 and Chapter 4).
- Procedures for changing or mixing supplies in distribution (see Section 3.5).
- Optimization of water treatment (including a full cost–benefit analysis) so that water entering the network is of good quality and the potential for regrowth in the network is minimized (see Chapter 2).
- Awareness of, and collaboration with, leakage reduction teams to identify where pressure reduction may result in low pressures.
- Good record keeping so that problems can be traced and lessons learnt. An electronic record is preferable for ease of storage and access.
- Collaboration with consumer services to keep consumers fully informed of activities on the network and any emergency advice in the case of a water quality problem (e.g. issuing boil water notices).

3.3 DESIGN AND OPERATION OF SERVICE RESERVOIRS

Service reservoirs (i.e. reservoirs that store treated water) allow fluctuations in demand to be accommodated without a loss of hydraulic integrity. They can also guarantee a supply, at least for part of the day, while the inflow into the network is stopped (e.g. for maintenance of the treatment works or upstream pipe, or a contamination incident).

Service reservoirs should be covered to avoid contamination of the water from animal faeces and other pollutants. Only covered reservoirs are considered here.

Using service reservoirs can allow the water to age by several hours (or days) and the disinfectant residual to decline, particularly in areas with high ambient temperatures. Regions of stagnant water are possible if the reservoir is not designed or operated correctly, and this creates a risk of poor-quality water entering the supply if the reservoir is operated outside its usual limits. Ingress of contaminants such as animal faeces is also a possibility (e.g. through poorly closing hatches, cracks in the walls and damaged vermin proofing).

There are two extremes of mixing in reservoirs: fully mixed and plug flow. In practice, the mixing will usually be between the two extremes (WRc, 1996). Fully mixed conditions are the preferred option for service reservoirs because the outlet disinfectant concentration with fully mixed conditions is better than that with plug flow. An exception is when disinfection is applied at the inlet for primary disinfection purposes, in which case plug flow is preferred, to allow sufficient contact time (as in the disinfection contact tank of a water treatment works).

Near fully mixed conditions are easier to achieve than near plug flow and there are fewer stagnant regions with fully mixed conditions than with an approximation to plug flow.

3.3.1 Shape and configuration

Service reservoirs can be in various forms; for example, towers and tanks (at ground level or underground). Towers provide the extra benefit of increasing pressure head to the downstream network, which is useful in flat regions. In situations where it is not critical to provide extra pressure above that provided by the geography of the land, then ground-level or underground tanks are sufficient. These can be placed on top of hills to use the natural pressure head.

The internal shape and configuration of a reservoir are major factors in maintaining water quality while the water is stored. The five subsections below describing important features of reservoirs summarize information from a report (WRc, 1996), which identifies the limitations and scope of application of these features.

Shape and dimension

As the ratio of length to breadth of a reservoir is increased, it becomes more difficult to achieve the (desirable) fully mixed condition. In the extreme case of a long, narrow reservoir, it would be necessary to place the inlet and outlet at opposite ends; the flow would then approximate to plug flow. Therefore, the reservoir should be circular or rectangular, with a low ratio of length to breadth. For new reservoirs without baffles, a length to breadth ratio of less than 2:1 is considered optimal for water quality. For existing reservoirs with a ratio greater than 2:1, it should still be possible to optimize water quality by minimizing the residence time (see Section 3.3.2) and noting the rules on inlet and depth.

Depth of water

Generally, in reservoirs without baffles, water quality is better where the average depth is greater than 3 m, because this facilitates mixing. However, in situations where a deep reservoir creates long residence times, a depth of less than 3 m may be a compromise design. A reservoir with an exceptionally large or small volume would have a different critical level, which would need to be determined for each case, using a technique such as computational fluid dynamics.

Inlet

As a guideline, in reservoirs without baffles, inlet velocities in excess of 0.1 m/s will promote the conditions desirable for optimal water quality. A turbulent jet is needed to ensure mixing. In reservoirs without baffles that meet the dimensions and depth considerations given above, there is no strong evidence for any one preferred inlet position. Inlet position is likely to be more important for cases outside the design and depth considerations given above. Computational fluid dynamic software can be used to determine the best inlet configuration (and service reservoir design generally). Positioning of inlets and outlets at opposite corners of the same wall (even if this is the shortest wall) is not detrimental to water quality in a well-mixed reservoir. Positioning of inlets and outlets closer than this should be avoided to minimize the risk of short-circuiting. In circular reservoirs, one particular inlet position (i.e. where the inlet has a horizontal flow parallel to the wall) is detrimental to water quality and should be avoided. Inlet velocity and position is less important for reservoirs with baffles, provided that the inlet is logically positioned at the beginning of the first baffle section.

Baffles

Generally, baffles should be avoided. When designing new reservoirs (that also meet the dimensional and depth ratios and inlet considerations above) the inclusion of baffles will give a worse water quality than if baffles are not used, especially where inlet flows are virtually continuous. For reservoirs with baffles, the inlet velocity and depth considerations given above would not improve water quality. However, the inclusion of compartments is worth considering (where each compartment is designed and operated as a separate service reservoir) for the operational advantage of being able to take individual compartments out of service for maintenance without affecting water supply.

Outlet

The outlet position is not critical in a well-mixed reservoir. Outlets need to be positioned on or near floor level in order to allow the full reservoir capacity to be used. Their position relative to the inlet is not as important as the above factors.

3.3.2 Flow pattern

The following aspects of flow pattern within a service reservoir may have a substantial effect on water quality (WRc, 1996).

Residence time

The factor that has the greatest overall effect on water quality is residence time, and this should be minimized to reduce both loss of disinfectant residual and the age of the water at the outlet. Minimizing residence time, within supplier or local requirements for security of supply, will improve water quality. As mentioned in Section 3.2.1, systems should not have excessive capacity unless an increase in future demand is probable.

Pumping and loss of supply

Long periods without pumping should be avoided. Short periods such as loss of inlet flow for several hours or where pumping is only at night may not cause poor water quality. What may be of concern is that such situations will cause variable disinfectant concentrations entering supply. Where intermittent pumping is unavoidable, baffles can be an advantage. In reservoirs with baffles, the variation in disinfectant during intermittent pumping is less marked. However, the need to control the disinfectant concentration should be balanced against the disadvantages of baffles (see Section 3.3.1).

Stratification

Where incoming water temperatures differ from those in the body of the reservoir, stratification can occur. This is only an issue in reservoirs with poor mixing because good mixing does not allow thermal strata to form. Stratification is undesirable because it promotes slower moving water in some parts of the reservoir, which could provide more opportunities for microbial growth.

3.3.3 General issues

Addressing the following general issues will also help maintain water quality in service reservoirs (also see Section 4.2).

Security of site

The potential for, and consequences of, contamination of the treated water in the reservoir are substantial. Service reservoirs should always be covered to prevent wildlife and people contaminating the water. Even if the reservoir is covered, all access points should be closed securely and checked regularly.

Risk assessment before operations

A risk assessment to identify potential problems and their consequences should be undertaken before any operations such as cleaning or seasonal use. Large numbers of people may be affected downstream of the reservoir if contamination occurs.

Sampling facilities

Sampling taps should be located to provide representative samples of water entering and leaving the reservoir. Sampling pipework should be constructed of material that does not support microbial growth (see Section 3.7) and kept to a minimum practical length. It is prudent to ensure that guidance on the minimum duration time for flushing the sampling pipework is provided at the sampling location.

Records

It is important that records are kept of the water quality, inlet and outlet flow rates, operations and any other activities that affect the reservoir. This provides an auditable trail in case of an incident, as well as valuable information for improving operations.

3.4 CONTROLLING DISINFECTANT RESIDUALS BY BOOSTER (RELAY) DOSING

3.4.1 Reasons for booster dosing

A disinfectant is typically added at the end of water treatment to give a disinfectant residual to provide some protection against microbial growth and limit the effects of contamination while the water is being conveyed through the distribution system. Chapter 2 (Section 2.3.1) for a discusses options for disinfectant residuals.

A disinfectant residual is normally consumed by exposed surfaces of materials in the network, deposits in the pipes, microorganisms and chemical species in the water (UKWIR, 2000c). It may also be consumed by contaminants entering the network; for example, as a result of cross-connections or backflow. Consequently, at the ends of long networks or networks with long transit times, the disinfectant residual concentration can be zero. This by itself is not a problem if there is no contamination or growth in microorganisms that would compromise either water quality or the monitoring of microbial quality. However, many water suppliers consider it prudent to maintain a residual to the extremities of the system, which may require disinfection stations within the network, a system known as "booster" or "relay" disinfection. (Note: maintaining the network (see Chapter 4) will help to maintain a disinfectant residual throughout the network, which may obviate the need for booster dosing.)

Design and operation   51

One method for maintaining a disinfectant residual throughout the network is to ensure a high residual concentration as water leaves the treatment works. However, this may mean that consumers immediately downstream of the treatment works receive concentrations of disinfectant that are undesirable because of tastes and odours. Booster disinfection provides an alternative solution.

3.4.2 Locating booster sites

Sampling water quality within a distribution system (at consumers' taps) will identify where the disinfectant residual is inadequate. It should be borne in mind that disinfectant residual will vary during the day as the demand, and hence transit times, change.

It would be a very expensive exercise to sample in sufficient density to assess the whole of a network. This is where water quality modelling software packages are valuable. Disinfectant residuals across the whole of the network can be modelled and areas where the disinfectant is likely to be inadequate identified. These software packages are extensions of hydraulic network models (see Section 3.2.1) where processes such as disinfectant residual decay in distribution can be modelled.

The models can also be used to test the suitability of sites for disinfection stations. By running the model, it is possible to gauge what disinfectant residual is needed at the potential sites to provide sufficient residual downstream as protection against microbial regrowth, taking into account the threshold for tastes and odours. The modelling may show that a particular site cannot be used because the disinfectant dose required to give sufficient residual concentration at downstream sites will cause taste and odour problems immediately downstream of the station.

The inlets and outlets of service reservoirs are common sites for booster disinfection. There are practical advantages: reservoirs usually provide a secure site and hence the dosing equipment can be installed in a safe environment where the public cannot easily gain access. Where a station is not on the supplier's property, then security and safety are key issues. It may be that the concern over security overrides all other considerations. Sites within the distribution system where equipment can be installed (see Section 3.4.3) may also be limited in number.

3.4.3 Equipment

Several types of equipment can be used for booster disinfection (WRc, 1995). Most are designed for use at remote sites. The following points should be considered when designing a relay station.

- *Pressure.* The pressure against which the dosing equipment needs to pump will influence the type of equipment that can be used.
- *Pump capacity.* The pump needs to operate in its mid-range when delivering the required dose. The dose needs to be appropriate for the water quality at the dosing station, the flow rate and the target disinfectant residual. Laboratory tests can be used to determine the disinfectant demand of the water and thus the required dose.
- *Volumetric versus flow-proportional dosing.* Flow-proportional dosing is the preferred option because it gives better control. A flow meter will be needed if flow-proportional dosing is adopted.
- *Feedback.* Control of dosing can be improved by using feedback from a disinfectant monitor. Such a system requires an online disinfectant monitor to provide a signal to the dosing pump. If the disinfectant concentration in the water before booster dosing is variable, feedback is important to ensure that the target disinfectant concentration is reached.
- *Maintenance.* Cost and frequency of equipment maintenance will affect staffing and budget requirements.
- *Power supply.* The power supply available (e.g. battery, mains, gravity, compressed air or solar) will influence the choice of both the equipment and the siting of the station.
- *Physical size of the equipment.* The location of the dosing equipment will impact on which equipment can be used and vice versa.
- *Reliability of the equipment.* The operating environment should be specified when selecting equipment.
- *Dosing.* Duplicate dosing arrangements are needed to provide security in case of a failure.
- *Liquid versus gaseous dosing chemicals.* Safety, cost and any by-products must be taken into account when deciding whether to use liquid or gaseous dosing chemicals.
- *Telemetry for online monitoring.* Access to a telemetry system will be required.

The equipment needs to be installed and maintained correctly to ensure that the disinfectant residual is kept at the required level. The equipment used should be fitted so that the disinfectant-solution feed pipe is fixed directly into the main or enters through a dedicated inlet on the service reservoir.

3.5 AVOIDING POTENTIAL PROBLEMS WHEN MIXING WATER SOURCES IN DISTRIBUTION

There are many distribution systems where waters from two or more sources mix within the network. In most cases this has no detrimental effect on water quality; however, if waters of significantly different composition mix in the system, quality problems may occur. It is therefore prudent to investigate potential problems before introducing a new source, and take corrective action where necessary. Those issues specific to microbial quality are dealt with in Section 3.5.3.

When an additional source is introduced, problems may occur in one or more of the following three general categories:

- Long-term change in the composition of water received by an area or by consumers — Some areas will receive water that differs from the previous supply. This may cause problems with certain industrial processes, destabilise pipe deposits and biofilms, and lead to complaints about aesthetic quality from consumers.
- Daily changes in the composition of the water received by an area or by consumers — Some parts of the network may receive water from different sources at different times of the day (tidal flow). Similar issues arise as with long-term change in composition, but in this case they are due to the short-term variability of the quality. These tidal flows are very difficult to manage.
- Blending of two different waters — Consumers may receive a blend of the two waters throughout the day. The ratio between the two waters may be constant or variable. Certain ratios may have greater detrimental effects than other ratios of the same waters, and some blends may even have effects that would not arise with either of the source waters alone.

3.5.1 Modelling and planning

Network models are a valuable way of investigating the effects of mixing. In particular, they can be used to predict where mixing will take place and how these locations vary with time of day, season and system operation. These questions can be answered with a hydraulic model, but water-quality modelling software has advantages in that it allows the source of water delivered to each point in the network to be determined; also, it can predict the proportion of water from each source delivered to each point at each time. These features enable the user to consider many of the issues raised in the previous section.

Expertise in the use of water-quality models is not as widespread as expertise with hydraulic models. Interpretation is more difficult, particularly in the area where mixing takes place. The mixing boundary itself is very sensitive to inaccuracies in the input data. The ratio of the mix at any point can also be sensitive to input values. Decisions should not be made on the assumption that results are accurate. It is prudent to carry out a sensitivity analysis and take action on the basis that a range of mixing boundaries and mixing ratios could occur in practice.

The available water-quality modelling software packages contain only limited process models. All the models handle the transport and blending of inert substances and the decay of disinfectant residual. Treatment of other parameters depends on the particular software package; however, microbiology is a particularly weak aspect of these programmes.

Laboratory testing provides an alternative to detailed modelling. Samples of the two waters can be mixed in the predicted proportions and determinations made of the relevant parameter values. Different consumers will receive different mixes and, as described above, there will usually be some error in the predicted blend. Therefore, a range of blends should be tested to determine the chemical and microbial changes that may occur and to identify the risks of introducing the new source.

It is important to realize that both the modelling and mixing tests will only predict the effects of the mixing process, not the effects related to the interactions with biofilms and other deposits in the network.

3.5.2 Introducing a new supply

Modelling and laboratory testing are described above in Section 3.5.1, which empasises the difficulty in producing accurate values for mixed parameters. Increased vigilance during the commissioning of a new supply is therefore recommended. Increased sampling may be necessary before, during and immediately after implementation. Sample points should be concentrated at the following locations:
- near to the predicted boundary between the areas supplied by the different waters;
- in areas supplied with a blend of different waters;
- in tidal flow areas where the source of the water changes during the day.

Samples should be analysed for parameters that the predictions have shown may be problematical. Sampling frequency and duration will depend on the nature of potential problems; if destabilisation of deposits is of concern, the effects could occur after a period of several weeks if not months.

Many complaints may be about the aesthetic quality of the water. While the water is safe, the different taste or appearance may be a cause of concern to consumers. Warning the affected consumers of the intended change and reassuring them of the water quality is an effective way to reduce complaints.

Some industrial users have very specific quality requirements. Consultation with users before implementation of change may demonstrate that there is no problem, or that the user can make simple process modifications to deal with the change.

3.5.3 Potential effects of mixing waters on disinfectant residual and microbial quality

Microbial growth in a water depends on temperature, nutrient content and disinfectant concentration. In a network, it will also depend on the composition of the internal pipe surfaces, but this effect cannot be predicted and is not discussed here. The temperature and nutrient content are relatively easy to predict in the mixed water because they will be the flow-weighted average of the values in the constituent waters. Disinfectant concentration will depend on the degree of decay in the constituent waters up to the point of mixing, the type of disinfectant in the constituent waters, the blending proportions and the chemical reactions between the disinfectant species. These are affected in turn by other compositional parameters such as pH of the mixed water.

If one source has not had its disinfectant demand satisfied and another source has a disinfectant residual, the combination of the two sources may result in the disinfectant demand of the mixed water being satisfied and the disinfectant residual concentration reducing to zero. This change will most readily be observed when surface waters and groundwaters are blended (WRc, 1990).

When the constituent waters contain different types of disinfectant, various scenarios can occur on mixing. Where the two disinfectants are free chorine and monochloramine, the reactions are complex and depend on the water composition (White, 1992).

Two of the possible effects that can occur when waters mix are described below (WRc, 1990).

- If a groundwater of good quality with a free chlorine residual of, for example, 0.2 mg/l, is mixed in equal volumes with another water with no chlorine residual but containing a relatively low concentration of ammonia (e.g. 0.02–0.04 mg/l ammonia-N), the ratio of chlorine to ammonia-N will favour the formation of dichloramine and nitrogen trichloride, both of which are ineffective disinfectants and cause taste and odour complaints.
- If the mixing of two waters produces a change in pH and the disinfectant is monochloramine, then monochloramine may convert to dichloramine. For example, at pH 8 only 5% dichloramine will be present, but at pH 7.5 the proportion would rise to 25%.

These examples emphasize the importance of undertaking laboratory mixing experiments before blending waters in distribution.

Low temperature and high disinfectant levels inhibit microbial growth, which otherwise depends on nutrient level. However, the relationships between growth and these controlling factors are not linear and it cannot be assumed that growth in a mixed water of equal proportions, for example, is midway between the growth in each of the constituent waters. Thus, a particular water may exhibit low microbial growth at low temperature and low disinfectant residual, as may another water at a higher temperature with a higher residual, but a mix of the two may support high microbial growth.

3.5.4 Changing flow conditions and existing deposits

Stable biofilms and other deposits may be disturbed by a change in flow conditions or by changes in water composition. A new source may radically change the flow pattern in parts of the network if the new point of entry is in a different location to the existing point of entry. Network modelling (see Section 3.5.1) is well suited to predicting these changes. Some pipes may have a large increase in flow rate or a change in flow direction, which may disturb deposits or strip biofilm from the pipe wall. This may have an adverse effect on the aesthetic and microbial quality of water at the consumer's tap.

Other pipes may contain water that has taken longer to reach this point than it did before the change (i.e. it is "older"). The water quality may thus be significantly different and the water may contain a higher concentration of disinfectant, leading to stripping of biofilm — a situation that can arise even if the new water entering the system is of the same quality as the existing supply.

The following changes in water composition often lead to destabilisation of deposits (WRc, 1990):

- changing from a hard (> 200 mg/l as calcium carbonate) to a very soft water (< 50 mg/l as calcium carbonate);
- a reduction in dissolved oxygen content of the conveyed water (a well-aerated supply has > 4 mg/l of oxygen);
- a substantial increase in dissolved organic content (low content is < 2 mg/l of carbon and high content is > 3 mg/l).

Although the effects of destabilised deposits are often temporary, it is recommended that networks are cleaned before a permanent change in water type or a substantial change in flow pattern (see Chapter 4).

3.6 POTENTIAL EFFECTS OF ZONING NETWORKS

3.6.1 Potential benefits

There are a number of reasons for dividing networks into zones but, essentially, the aim is to achieve greater control over the distribution of water. An example is the practice of dividing the network into "district meter areas" for leakage control purposes, where valves are closed so that a group of 1000–2000 properties is supplied through a single flow meter. Whatever the prime reason for zoning, there are potential benefits from a water quality standpoint.

- Containment of water quality incidents (e.g. contamination) is much easier if an area can be rapidly isolated. If the zone is small, then it should be possible to contain the problem in a small area.
- Zoning can reduce the extent and complexity of mixing in distribution so that more consumers are regularly supplied with the same water quality; the problems described in Section 3.5 are therefore minimized.
- Interpretation of sample analysis data is easier.

3.6.2 Potential disadvantages

Zoning can improve water quality in some parts of the network and reduce quality in others (UKWIR, 2000b). Creating a zone changes the flow pattern in the network. Some pipes will have increased flow velocity, possibly resuspending deposits, and others will have decreased flow velocity, possibly allowing deposition. The age of the water when it reaches some properties will be less and, at other points, more. At properties where the age of the water has increased substantially, water quality may deteriorate.

Although some consumers will benefit and others suffer from the change, it is possible to limit the extent of the deleterious effects by careful siting of the closed valves. Of particular concern is the creation of new dead-ends with zero flow or long lengths with very low flow. Water quality close to the closed valve can become particularly poor and there will be increased deposition from the slow moving water.

Dead-ends are particularly important when the boundary valves are opened. On these occasions, poor-quality water will be carried into the zone or into the neighbouring zone. It is good practice to clean the dead-end lengths on each side of the boundary valve before the valve is opened. Washouts installed close to the valve on each side will facilitate this process.

3.6.3 Implementing changes

Before implementation, it is important to identify risks so that, if necessary, designs can be modified, consumers informed and remedial action planned.

58   Safe Piped Water

Network modelling is a useful tool for predicting the effect of zoning on velocities, disinfectant concentration and age of water. Where low disinfectant concentration, long times of travel or long lengths of near-stagnant water are predicted, it may be possible to improve the situation by changing the valve positions. Models can also be used to identify the effect of the design changes or remedial measures. For example, booster disinfection may be needed because zoning will lead to low concentrations in part of the network. The best site and required set point for a disinfection station can be determined using a network model (see Section 3.4 for more details on booster dosing).

It is prudent to increase sampling in the period before, during and immediately after rezoning, as for the introduction of a new supply (see Section 3.5.2).

3.7 PIPE MATERIALS

Treated water conveyed through a piped network is exposed to numerous surfaces. It is important that no materials placed in contact with the drinking-water in the network promote microbial growth or leach any contaminants into the water that can support microbial growth (see the WHO companion text *Managing the Safety of Materials and Chemicals Used in the Production and Distribution of Drinking-water*, in preparation).

A materials approval system, where materials are tested to see if they meet defined standards before they can be added to a list of approved materials, is a recommended approach. There is no universally accepted system for such approvals. Some countries have their own national approval scheme (NAS), others leave the selection of safe materials to the individual water supply organizations.

Most approval schemes are based on tests where the product is kept in contact with test water under specified test conditions. Various tests are undertaken to assess whether the material, or contaminants arising from the material, can:
- adversely affect general water quality;
- exceed permissible levels set in national standards and positive lists, etc;
- pose a health risk to consumers.

These schemes may or may not address the ability of the materials to support or promote microbial growth. Details are beyond the scope of this review but a summary of the European approval systems and the development of a harmonized European acceptance scheme is available (WRc-NSF, 2001). The USA approval systems are based on plumbing codes and standards set by the American National Standards Institution and NSF (www.nsf.org).

The condition of existing materials in the network is also important and this is addressed in Chapter 4.

3.8 PIPE LOCATION

Water mains should be installed using adequate separation from potential sources of contamination such as sewers, storm water pipes, pipes carrying reclaimed wastewater and drainage fields for septic tanks. The appropriate separation will depend on pipe material and joint type, soil conditions and space for repair (AWWARF, 2001). Local recommendations should be followed. For example, the following separation distances are recommended in certain USA standards (Great Lakes, 1997):
- a 3 m horizontal separation between water mains and sanitary sewer force mains or sewers installed in parallel;
- a 45.7 cm vertical separation for a water main crossing above or below a sewer or force main.

3.9 PROTECTION FROM CROSS-CONNECTION AND BACKFLOW AT POINT OF DELIVERY

3.9.1 Sanitary significance

Piped water supplies are vulnerable to contamination at the point of delivery to consumers, which may be domestic households, institutions or premises for commerce, agriculture and industry. At these locations, water is transferred within the property and used not only for consumption via a tap but stored in tanks or supplied to various equipment. The water supply organization has less effective control of pipework in these situations than in the main supply network. There is a potential for backflow of water from these premises into the mains network. This may be driven by high pressures generated in equipment connected to mains water supplies, or by low pressures in the mains as described previously in this chapter. A backflow event will be a sanitary problem if there is cross-connection between the potable supply and a source of contamination. A cross-connection can be defined as: "any actual or potential connection or structural arrangement between a public or private potable water system and any other source or system though which it is possible to introduce into any part of the potable system any used water, industrial fluids, gas or substance other than the intended potable water with which the potable system is supplied" (USC FCCCHR, 1993). Examples of potential sources of cross-connections include beverage dispensers, garden hose sprayers, water jetting equipment and fire sprinkling systems. Reviews of waterborne disease outbreaks in municipal systems often identify backflow events as a causative factor. In the USA, drinking-water contamination from backflow events has caused more waterborne disease outbreaks than any other factor (Dyksen, 1997; Craun, 1981).

3.9.2 Cross-connection control

Controlling cross-connections and preventing backflow depends on factors that are largely governed by the legal aspects of water supply in a particular country. Normally, at some point on the system the responsibility for the pipework will transfer from supplier to property owner. This is where protection for the potable water supply distribution system (e.g. a backflow prevention device installed in conjunction with a stop valve and meter) may be installed if considered necessary. The location is usually in a protected but accessible place near the boundary of the consumer's property. The consumer's system downstream of this point may contain potentially hazardous cross-connections. It may be the property owner's responsibility to identify hazards and provide those individual connections with backflow prevention devices to protect the potable water system within the property. Ideally, the backflow protection devices should be registered with the water supplier and should comply with a standard procedure for assessing the hazard.

Requirements for protection from contamination of pressurized potable water systems at cross-connection points are normally set out in appropriate regulations and adopted by the local or national legislature. The water supply agency or the appropriate governing body then implements these regulations. Cross-connection regulations will typically include the following measures (AWWA, 1990; AS/NZS, 1998):

- definition of responsibilities for cross-connection control;
- identification of personnel to perform inspections;
- categorization of cross-connection hazards and appropriate devices for each level of hazard;
- inspection schedules;
- records of control devices maintained in the system;
- procedures for installing devices on new constructions;
- details of requirements for devices to prevent backflow, in terms of materials, design, performance (including air gaps and break tanks), field testing and maintenance;
- education and certification programmes for employees;
- education programmes for the public on the hazards of cross-connections and devices that can be used in the home.

Box 3.2. An outbreak of Giardiasis at a campsite.

During the summer of 1979, an estimated 1850 people became ill with diarrhoea after camping at a private campsite in Arizona. Of seven stool samples examined, six were positive for *Giardia duodenalis*. Drinking-water from a tap on the site was implicated as the cause of the outbreak following a postal questionnaire. Of 53 people who said they had drunk the water, 51 (96%) reported illness, compared to only 3 of 12 who had not drunk it (25%). There was also a significant dose response relationship between the amount of water drunk and the risk of illness.

The water system on the site had been developed over a period of six years under the management of four separate owners. Records covering the design and maintenance of the water supply system were not available. Drinking-water came from a shallow well and was pumped to a storage tank above the campsite. The campground had its own sewage system. On investigation, it was found that both the drinking-water and sewage system used pipes of the same type and colour. Both systems operated under pressure, with the pressure in the sewage system being greater than in the drinking-water system.

Although water samples had been collected for bacteriological analysis on neighbouring sites, none had been taken from the implicated site until the outbreak. Of 11 samples taken after the outbreak was detected, three had very high coliform counts. These three samples were taken from taps that had been associated with increased risk of illness in the epidemiological study.

When fluorescein dye was introduced into the sewage treatment plant, the tap water became intensely coloured. Excavation of the distribution system revealed a direct connection between the sewage and drinking-water systems. This outbreak illustrates the importance of:

- maintaining adequate records of the design and maintenance of water and sewage systems;
- using clearly different markings to indicate drinking-water and sewerage systems;
- routine microbiological monitoring of all water supply systems.

Source: Starko et al. (1986).

Typical definitions for degrees of cross-connection hazard ratings are as follows:
- *High hazard* — Any condition, device or practice that, in connection with the potable water supply system, has the potential to cause death.
- *Medium hazard* — Any condition, device or practice that, in connection with the potable water supply system, could endanger health.
- *Low hazard* — Any condition, device or practice that, in connection with the potable water supply system, would constitute a nuisance but would not endanger health or cause injury.

The type of backflow prevention device installed has to be consistent with the hazard rating.

3.9.3 Backflow prevention devices

There are various types of backflow prevention devices; those listed below are the more common.

Air gap

An air gap is the most basic protection measure where potable water can flow without any possibility of a backflow, siphon or pressurized return of used water or contaminated substance. An air gap is suitable for use in high, medium or low-hazard conditions. A simple example is the sink inlet valve or tap, with its discharge point well above the overflow level of water in the sink.

Break tank

The air gap principle is extended to create a new supply head (pressure) and, if the tank is allowed to overflow, an air gap is maintained to the water inlet. The break tank provides a separated supply system that effectively isolates the potable water supply system from a new gravity head or a source for a pumped supply. A break tank is suitable for use in high, medium or low-hazard conditions. A simple example is the float-valve controlled toilet flushing cistern.

Mechanical control valves

Mechanical control valves are subject to wear and eventual failure. An inspection and maintenance programme is usually required, with the results of the programme to be reported to the water supplier. The following are types of mechanical backflow prevention devices that are typically installed downstream of the meter or stop valve at the property boundary. (There are other types designed for special operational conditions.)

- *The dual check valve (dual CV).* This valve is designed for use in low-hazard conditions. The device is nontestable and is typically installed in domestic or residential water services. The dual CV consists of two independently acting nonreturn valves in series, arranged to be force loaded in the closed position. Domestic or residential basic size water meters are available with a dual CV included. The combination (water meter plus dual CV) is cheaper to purchase than the two components individually.
- *The double check valve (double CV).* This valve is designed for use in medium-hazard conditions. This is a testable device and is typically used in smaller industrial or commercial water services. The double CV consists of two independently acting nonreturn valves in series, arranged to be force loaded in the closed position. Three test taps are included on the double CV, (upstream, intermediate and downstream) to enable regular checking of the valve performance. These devices are usually designed to allow the valves to be replaced without removing the device from the pipeline assembly.
- *The double check detector assembly (DCDA).* This assembly is also designed for use in medium-hazard conditions. This is a testable device intended for use with fire services; it allows monitoring or metering of small draw-off of water for general use within the property. The DCDA consists of a double CV or a pair of nonreturn valves, a by-pass line with isolating ball valves and test taps, water meter and secondary double CV.
- *The reduced pressure zone assembly (RPZA).* This assembly is designed for use in high-hazard conditions. This is a testable device and is typically used in industrial water services. The RPZA consists of two independently acting nonreturn valves in series, arranged to be force loaded in the closed position; and a relief valve positioned between the nonreturn valves, force loaded to be open to the atmosphere whenever the pressure differential across the upstream nonreturn valve reduces to a specified amount. Test taps are also provided for performance checking.

3.9.4 Typical property hazard ratings

Hazard ratings for different property types are useful for designating the type of cross-connection protection required. A qualified person nominated or approved by the regulating body should assess each connection. Table 3.1 provides some typical hazard ratings by type of connection.

Table 3.1. Typical hazard ratings for different types of connection.[a]

Type of connection	Hazard rating
Agricultural, horticultural and general chemical processes	High
Buildings with recirculating water air-conditioning systems	High
Factories using toxic chemicals and processing water other than potable water	High
Hospitals, mortuaries and veterinary clinics	High
Industrial or commercial cleaning processes	High
Food preparation and beverage processing plants	Medium
High rise buildings	Medium
Hotels and large apartment blocks with swimming pool	Medium
Public swimming pools	Medium
Secondary schools with laboratories	Medium
Individual residential premises (typical)	Low
Small apartment blocks (typical)	Low
Industrial or commercial buildings	As assessed

Source: AS/NZS 3500.1.2:1998

3.9.5 Field testing and maintenance of backflow protection devices

Registered air gaps and break tanks should comply with the dimensions specified in regulations. Mechanical backflow prevention devices used for high and medium hazards should comply with the manufacturing and performance requirements nominated in regulations. For high and medium-rated hazards, the dimensions and function of each installation should be independently inspected and tested for operation by a qualified person after installation. Typical regulations specify testing after maintenance or repair and regularly at intervals not exceeding 12 months.

Service connections for residential properties and smaller commercial premises usually attract a low-hazard rating, and water suppliers may not have considered backflow prevention devices an important issue for these connections. However, some service connections use a stop tap incorporating a nonreturn valve that acts as a backflow prevention device. In some cases, the connections are fitted with two stop taps, one at the water main tapping (connection) and another at the meter. These stop taps effectively represent the performance equivalent of a dual CV. The backflow protection function of these valves cannot be tested for operation without shut down and removal, which is an unlikely event. It is not unusual for many of these connections to be in service for decades without any inspection or maintenance, and it could be expected that backflow prevention would not be effective in time. Instead of stop taps, some supply systems are connected using ball valves that have no backflow prevention capacity. The water company may rely on the meter for backflow prevention because the basic meter is designed to include at least one nonreturn valve.

Where water by measure (metered service) is used as the predominant method of payment to the water company and the meter is used to provide backflow protection, renewal of the meter will also ensure renewal of the backflow prevention device. Many governments and regulators are legislating for accuracy in measurement for public metered systems, which results in more regular meter replacement by water companies. The performance of different types of water meters can be modelled by the water company under the varied operational conditions encountered. The model includes operational costs and income received, and an economic meter renewal period can be established. Water meters containing a dual CV provide water agencies with the opportunity to replace both at a prescheduled time.

3.10 HEALTH RELATED DESIGN AND OPERATIONS CHECKLIST

Pipe network

- Set minimum pressures to prevent intrusion and provide adequate flows at all delivery points in the distribution network.
- Maintain pressure in the network within a maximum that avoids pipe breaks and a minimum that supplies adequate flow rates to meet expected demands.
- Minimize low-flow dead-ends and loops to prevent water "stagnation".
- Do not design with excessive capacity unless required to meet a known increase in future demand.
- Avoid situations that may give rise to negative pressures. Hydraulic models can be used to identify where these may occur and to identify solutions.
- Install nonreturn valves on the supply inlet to premises where high back pressures could be accidentally generated.
- Incorporate fixtures and designs that facilitate maintenance with minimum disruption to normal flow regimes and that prevent the ingress of contaminants at low pressures.
- Prevent pressure surges by controlling the switching of pumps and the operation of the valves. Use surge analysis to plan antisurge techniques.
- Where possible, avoid the use of pressure relief valves, double acting air valves and surge shafts to relieve surge because they may allow ingress of contaminants.

- In intermittent supplies, identify particularly high-risk areas and reduce hazards. Give high priority to preventing intermittence.
- Perform risk assessments of all operational activities that may affect water quality and ensure that documented procedures are used by all those that are involved.

Service reservoirs

- Cover service reservoirs to prevent contamination.
- Ensure that all hatches and structures are secure and vermin proof.
- Ensure that sampling facilities will provide representative samples.
- Use fully-mixed flow if possible; consider the effect of shape, dimensions and inlet conditions on the residence time and flow pattern in the reservoir.
- Perform risk assessments of all operational activities that may affect water quality and ensure that documented procedures are used by all those involved.
- Keep records of all activities on, and information about, the reservoirs.

Controlling disinfectant residuals

- Use booster dosing within distribution to avoid excessive doses at the start of the network to achieve a residual at the extremities.
- Use hydraulic models to help in identifying suitable locations.
- Ensure secure location of booster equipment.
- Consider the effects of mixing different water sources in distribution, or changing the water supply, on the resulting disinfectant residuals.

Zoning networks

- Select boundaries to minimize dead-ends and water transit times, and to maintain pressures.
- Select boundaries to aid the containment of water contamination incidents and the monitoring of parameters of hygienic significance.
- Install washouts either side of boundary valves to clean out dead-end lengths before opening boundary valves.
- Consider whether deposits may be disturbed by changes in flow velocity and direction.

Materials of construction and pipe location

- Adopt a materials approval scheme that prevents the use of materials that may promote microbial growth (or may pose any other health risk to consumers).

- When installing water mains, ensure adequate separation from potential sources of contamination such as sewers, storm water pipes, pipes carrying reclaimed wastewater and drainage fields for septic tanks.

Cross-connections and backflow
- Inform the public (and plumbers) about the hazards of cross-connections, their responsibilities and the control devices that can be used in the home.
- Specify a hazard rating system and backflow prevention devices for each level of hazard.
- Adopt a policy for testing and maintenance of backflow protection devices according to hazard rating and risk.

3.11 SUMMARY

Water supply organizations should adopt network design and operating strategies that prioritize issues closely linked to water supply hygiene. In particular, such strategies should specify how the organization would:
- identify and prevent low pressures, especially negative pressures, in the system;
- prevent pressure surges in the network;
- design the network to minimize the risks of contamination during operational activities and to avoid water stagnation;
- design and operate service reservoirs to avoid contamination by ingress and to avoid stagnation;
- control disinfectant residuals in distribution systems;
- assess the effect of different supplies entering the network;
- determine the benefits and problems of zoning the network;
- select construction materials that do not promote microbial growth;
- prevent cross-connections and backflow.

3.12 REFERENCES

AS/NZS (1998). Australian and New Zealand Standard AS/NZS 3500.1.2:1 *National plumbing and drainage code. Part 1.2: water supply — acceptable solutions.* (http://www.standards.com.au).

AWWA (1990). *Manual M14: recommended practice for backflow protection and cross-connection control.* American Water Works Association, USA.

AWWARF (2001). *Pathogen intrusion into the distribution system.* American Water Works Association Research Foundation, Denver, USA, 72.

Craun GF (1981). Outbreaks of waterborne disease in the United States: 1971–1978. *Journal of the American Water Works Association*, 73(7):360–369.

Dyksen J (1997). Issue paper no. 4 — Distribution system reliability. In: *Managerial assessment of water quality and system reliability.* American Water Works Association Research Foundation, Denver, USA.

Great Lakes Upper Mississippi River Board of State Public Health and Environmental Managers (1997). *Recommended standards for water works.* Health Education Services, Albany, New York.

LeChevallier MW et al. (2003). The potential for health risks from intrusion of contaminants into the distribution system from pressure transients. *Journal of Water and Health,* 1(1):3–14.

Morse LJ et al. (1972). The Holy Cross College football team hepatitis outbreak. *Journal of the American Medical Association,* 219:706–708.

OFWAT (1999). *July return — reporting requirements and definitions manual.* Office of Water Services, Birmingham, UK.

Starko KM et al. (1986). Campers' diarrhea outbreak traced to water-sewage link. *Public Health Reports*; 101:527–31.

UKWIR (2000a). *Operational and maintenance strategies for maintaining water quality in distribution systems.* Report 00/DW/03/12, UK Water Industry Research Limited, London.

UKWIR (2000b). *Effect of district meter areas on water quality.* Report 00/DW/03/13, UK Water Industry Research Limited, London.

UKWIR (2000c). *Toolboxes for maintaining and improving drinking water quality.* Report 00/DW/03/11, UK Water Industry Research Limited, London.

USC FCCHR (1993). University of Southern California, Foundation for Cross-Connection Control and Hydraulic Research. *Manual of Cross-Connection Control, 9th Edition.* Los Angeles, California, USA.

Webber NB (1971). *Fluid mechanics for civil engineers.* Chapman and Hall, London.

White GC (1992). *Handbook of chlorination and alternative disinfectants,* 3rd ed. Van Nostrand Reinhold, New York.

WRc (1990). *Aesthetic water quality problems in distribution systems. A source document for the water mains rehabilitation manual.* WRc plc, Swindon, UK.

WRc (1995). *Final report: controlled release principles and materials for preventing microbiological failures: Part 1 — review of existing and novel technology for boosting disinfectant residual.* Report PT 1061, WRc plc, Swindon, UK.

WRc (1996). *Final report: operation and design of potable water reservoirs.* Report PT 2018, WRc plc, Swindon, UK.

WRc (2000). *The effects of system operation on water quality in distribution.* Report PT 2095, WRc plc, Swindon, UK.

WRc–NSF (2001). *European approval systems. Effects of materials on water quality,* 2nd ed. WRc–NSF Ltd, Medmenham, UK.

Wylie EB, Streeter VL (1978). *Fluid transients,* McGraw-Hill.

4
Maintenance and survey of distribution systems

Dammika Vitanage, Francis Pamminger and Tony Vourtsanis

4.1 INTRODUCTION

Previous chapters have discussed:
- design of pipework and associated facilities to prevent contamination
- system operation to maintain pressure and structural integrity
- design and operation to avoid stagnation and preserve water quality
- prevention of deposits and biofilm by good water treatment.

Succeeding chapters provide guidance on sanitary practices for repairs and construction, and advice on the effects of small animals proliferating in the network. Achieving the objectives given in each of these chapters depends on the distribution system being well maintained and in good structural condition.

© 2004 World Health Organization. *Safe Piped Water: Managing Microbial Water Quality in Piped Distribution Systems*. Edited by Richard Ainsworth. ISBN: 1 84339 039 6. Published by IWA Publishing, London, UK.

This chapter discusses maintenance and survey procedures that should form part of a water safety plan (see Chapter 7). It looks first at procedures that are applied to readily accessible features such as service reservoirs or valves, and then at procedures applied to the inside of pipework, where condition is inferred from water quality measurements or by inspection, which may be difficult.

In many older systems the condition of the pipework may have deteriorated to such an extent that targeted renovation and replacement is necessary to maintain operability. This can occur where iron pipes have corroded internally to produce hard encrustations that prevent the maintenance of water pressure and disinfectant residuals, or where external corrosion and ground movement have created excessive leakage. Such situations obviously require careful investigation to identify the appropriate engineering solution. This process is usually called rehabilitation planning (Evins et al., 1989; AWWA, 2001) and it incorporates more complex and costly methods than those used for planned maintenance and survey. Rehabilitation planning is not covered in this review, except in this chapter, where there are references to common approaches (e.g. selection of pipe-cleaning methods).

4.2 MAINTENANCE AND SURVEY OF RESERVOIRS, TANKS AND FITTINGS

4.2.1 Sanitary significance

Structural deficiencies in tanks and reservoirs may lead to the direct contamination of water supplies with pathogens. Also, sediments may form in tanks and reservoirs due to the relatively low flow velocities that are a feature of these structures. Although such sediments are unlikely to be of direct health significance, they make it difficult to maintain a disinfectant residual. If the water level of the reservoir drops rapidly, accumulated sediments can be drawn into the pipework, where they are difficult to remove and have an even greater effect on disinfectant residual and general microbial activity than in the reservoir.

Faulty seals, joints or connections on valves, hydrants and washouts may also allow contamination of the system. This is unlikely if the system is operating at design pressures because the leakage flow will be from the pipe outwards. However, low or negative pressures may draw in contamination. The occurrence of low and negative pressures can be extensive during emergencies. For example, surge modelling on three well-operated systems in the USA demonstrated that conditions such as the loss of pumping power, fire flow and pipe breaks created low or negative pressures at up to nearly 30% of the pipe intersection points (nodes) incorporated in the models (AWWARF, 2001).

Where supplies are intermittent, contamination is likely to occur, and it may be difficult to operate the system to reduce the risks of backflow. In managing risks from intermittent supplies, it is important to reduce the hazards that may cause contamination and the risks of ingress of water contaminated with faecal material. Reducing intermittence will require careful analysis of both the causes and the solutions. The management of water demand and the implementation of water conservation measures such as hosepipe bans can provide rapid, long-lasting solutions. However, these measures may be insufficient where the infrastructure needs to be reinforced (e.g. by providing storage tanks and service reservoirs), or repaired, to prevent leakage and wastage in the distribution system.

4.2.2 Service reservoirs and tanks

Table 4.1 provides a typical checklist for external examination of reservoirs to identify potential sanitary deficiencies.

The frequency of internal inspection and cleaning of a reservoir will depend on the rate of deposition of solids, the effect of the solids on water quality and the construction, age and ground characteristics. In many systems, inspection and cleaning will require detailed planning to minimize disruption to supplies and to avoid contamination. Detailed advice is available (Tarbet, Thomas & Brown, 1993). It is vital to observe safety and hygiene requirements during inspection and during any cleaning that is performed. The appropriate safety measures for working in confined spaces should be followed. Minimum hygienic conditions for reservoir entry should include facilities for disinfecting boots, gloves and equipment. These may include foot baths with disinfectant solution and the provision of clean disinfected mats around the hatch. It is also advisable to provide toilet facilities on site. General guidelines about the use of personnel in situations where they could contaminate water supplies are given in Section 5.3. Table 4.2 provides a typical checklist for the internal examination of reservoir structures to identify deficiencies of potential sanitary significance.

Table 4.1. A checklist for the external examination of reservoirs.

Item	Check
Grounds and banks	Trees, bushes and scrub close to reservoir; localized luxuriant growth of grass (indicative of leakage); wet patches; animal damage; cracks and signs of ground movement
Roof cover	Cracks, animal damage or ponding indicative of poor drainage
Roofing membrane	Where visible check for damage, de-bonding and cracks (especially at joins and edges)
Hatches	Damage to cover, lock, built-in ventilators and seals
Ventilators	Corrosion, dents, cracks, vandalism, integrity and suitability of the mesh, excessive number of ventilators
Overflow or washout	Operability or existence of the flap valve, corrosion of flap valve and pipe, condition of discharge point, protection from backflow and intrusion by vermin
Valve housing or chamber	Security, leakage from reservoir, operability of valves if possible, corrosion of valves, leakage from valves, labelling
Valve gear, telemetry, gauges	All points where cables or spindles pass through into the reservoir
Disinfection system	Security of housing and operation of the equipment

Source: Tarbet, Thomas & Brown (1993).

Table 4.2. A checklist for the internal examination of reservoirs.

Item	Check
Valves	Corrosion and operability, washout blockages.
Pipework	Corrosion, fixings, outlet screens and outlet blockages
Roof, walls and floor	Roof to wall joints, locations where spindles, hatches etc pass through the roof, indications of leakage such as stains and deposits, root intrusion and cracks
Deposits	Depth and location, take samples for analysis

Source: Tarbet, Thomas & Brown (1993).

Cleaning of internal surfaces

Certain aspects of the internal inspection normally require the internal surfaces to be cleaned and freed of deposits. Pressure jetting and chemical cleaning are the two methods commonly used for this.

Pressure-jet washing employs specialized equipment; it may damage weak surfaces and coatings, and expose aggregate on concrete surfaces. Therefore, the jetting pressure should be selected and tested with care, and provisions made for localized repairs. Following jetting, surfaces should be sprayed with a disinfecting solution. A typical solution contains 10–20 mg/l of free chlorine.

Any chemical cleaning system that is used should be suitable for a potable water system. Those that have been employed consist of a dilute solution of hypochlorous acid, or a dilute solution of organic or inorganic acids plus vitamin C (ascorbic acid). Provided the manufacturer's instructions are followed, these chemical cleaning methods should not damage the structure. Whichever method is employed, there will be a requirement to dispose of the deposits, disinfecting solutions and cleaning solutions in an environmentally acceptable manner.

Alternative inspection and cleaning methods may be available, based on diving equipment or robot-based technology. When using these techniques for inspection there are potential advantages of reduced disruption to reservoir operation and safer working conditions. However, if they are being considered for cleaning, then the difficulties of removing packed sediments and effectively disinfecting walls could be a disadvantage.

Frequency of inspection and cleaning

Many water supply organizations undertake the inspection and cleaning of service reservoirs at 1–5 year intervals, depending on factors such as water-quality measurements, the efficiency of water treatment in removing deposit-forming substances, the presence of animals and information from previous inspections.

External sanitary surveys may be undertaken more frequently, using standardized forms designed for the specific reservoir. These surveys should focus particularly on sanitary and structural integrity, and any obvious deviations from good operational practice such as inundated valves, inspection covers left open and damaged vent-pipe mesh. Routine visitors to the reservoir should be encouraged to report any visible defects promptly and operational staff should respond rapidly to identified problems. Where operators visit service reservoirs daily, they should be given the task of regular inspection of the reservoir.

4.2.3 Valves and other fittings

Valves are used to isolate and control flow, regulate pressure or prevent backflow. A range of valve types exists, with various design features to achieve different operating requirements.

The most common valve function in a distribution system is to isolate flow, by being either open or shut. Valves at the boundaries of supply zones are shut to maintain a specific pressure within a supply zone, whereas those within a supply zone are generally open. Thus, valves could be in the same operational position for long periods. Distribution valves assist the operation of a water-supply system at times of pipe failures, supply deficiencies, seasonal supply changes and mains cleaning. Their predominant function is to isolate sections or to configure the systems differently to maintain supply. Thus, having all valves locatable and operable is important in minimizing the number of consumers affected during both emergencies and planned maintenance.

Hydrants provide fire authorities with access to sufficient water in case of a fire, and can be used for air release at high points. In practice, hydrants are used for a number of other reasons, such as flushing mains to improve water quality, and filling water trucks and street sweepers. Above-ground hydrants are easier to see, which is useful to fire authorities at critical times. However, placing hydrants below ground avoids the potential for vehicular accidents and reduces the chance of vandalism. Washouts are fittings designed to drain and aid the flushing of mains; they are usually located at the ends of mains or low points along a pipeline.

These valves and other fittings are important for the efficient operation of the system to maintain water quality. They are also potential points of ingress for contaminants, including pathogens. If a burst occurs or there are unusual demands, low or negative pressures may allow ingress through sealing mechanisms. Valves and other fittings should therefore be regularly inspected and maintained to meet the following requirements (Walski, 1994):

- the type and location of all fittings are accurately recorded;
- valves and fittings are accessible and boxes are not buried under asphalt or paved over;
- valve and fittings boxes are clear of debris, well drained and show no signs of leakage;
- valves and fittings are in operable condition, and sealing mechanisms are in good order;
- valves are in the intended position (either open or shut);
- the turning direction and required number of turns for all valves is known.

Exercising or operating valves requires skill and care. It is possible to open or shut valves too quickly, causing surge, which can lead to main breaks or low pressures. Valves that have not been operated for a long time can break if too much pressure is applied. Operation of such valves can also dislodge rust and sediments, adversely affecting water quality. Closing such valves may also be complicated if sediments lodge in the valve seat, requiring operation of a nearby hydrant to dislodge these sediments. It is important that only suitably trained personnel operate valves.

Box 4.1. An outbreak of Norwalk viral gastroenteritis due to backflow between a septic tank and the water supply.

During May 1978, an outbreak of gastroenteritis affected staff and students at a school in Pierce County, Washington State, USA. The main clinical features were nausea, vomiting and abdominal pain. Two of three people from whom paired sera were collected showed a fourfold rise in titre to Norwalk virus. The attack rate in the school was 71.5%, compared to only 6.5% in a control school. There was a very strong correlation between illness and reporting consumption of tap water in the school. Furthermore, two soccer teams from other schools met at the school and players from these teams who drank water were 14 times more likely to be ill than those who did not drink the water.

The water supply to the school came from a 51 m deep well yielding 257 l/m. The water was not chlorinated. The school was not connected to the public sewer and used a septic tank. Well water was pumped to a pressure tank through a ball-check release valve, with the pressure being maintained by on–off cycling of the pump. When the pump switched off, a port in the valve opened to allow air into the system. This air was expelled when the pump switched on again. At this point, it was common for water to spill out of the valve and maintenance staff had therefore attached a pipe from the valve to a floor drain. On 2 May, a baffle to the septic tank blocked and foul water filled the boiler room floor to a depth of 20 cm, completely covering the end of the pipe from the ball-check release valve.

As soon as the outbreak was identified, maintenance staff took samples from five taps in the school and all five showed thermotolerant (faecal) coliforms. It was concluded that the drinking-water had become contaminated with foul water through the pipe from the release valve that had aspirated water up the pipe.

Source: Taylor, Gary & Greenberg (1981).

4.3 MAINTENANCE AND SURVEY OF PIPES

4.3.1 Sanitary significance

Externally-derived pathogens can potentially persist within deposits in a pipeline (see Section 1.3.3), and can present an underlying health concern if resuspended with the deposits and then consumed. Although there are no reports of health effects directly attributed to this mechanism, maintaining the internal cleanliness of the network is a prudent objective. Deposits provide an environment for the proliferation of microorganisms and animals, which may make the water unpalatable. This may result in consumers turning to alternative potentially unsafe sources, and may also make it difficult to identify contamination of hygienic significance by routine monitoring. The deposits also hinder the maintenance of a disinfectant residual, especially in the smaller diameter pipes, which are at greatest risk of low pressures and hence contamination.

4.3.2 Strategies for pipe networks
The most important problems associated with networks are:
- hygienic water-quality problems
- aesthetic water-quality problems
- hydraulic deficiencies
- structural performance problems
- leakage.

Hygienic water-quality problems are clearly the most important of these; however, identifying the best solution requires information about the other problems. This can be a complex process because of the variety of pipe materials and pipe ages usually found in a network, and the fact that a relatively small part of a pipeline may be responsible for a problem.

Many utilities have found that a programme of regular mains cleaning to remove loose deposits and animal infestations has been of great assistance in maintaining water quality in distribution. A range of activities and solutions may be available, such as simple flushing of selected pipe lengths, swabbing, relining pipes with either structural or nonstructural linings and mains renewal. The costs and complexity of these are obviously different and dictate that problems are investigated in a systematic way based on performance data. These strategic investigation and planning procedures, which should also consider the future demands on the system, are beyond the scope of this review. Representative methodologies for systematic rehabilitation planning have been published (Evins, Liebeschuetz & Williams, 1989; AWWA, 2001; Lei & Sægrov, 1998; Herz, 1998).

Three methods are generally used to clean pipes; flushing, air scouring and swabbing with compressible foam swabs. These methods are often referred to as nonaggressive techniques. An important attribute is that they can be used without having to cut into the mains and are therefore suitable for regular maintenance. Some cleaning methods (e.g. pressure jetting, mechanical scraping and abrasive swabs) do require cutting into mains and, if the pipe material is ferrous, also require subsequent relining of the pipe. Complexities like this require systematic rehabilitation planning.

Programmes of regular mains cleaning should not become a substitute for efficient treatment (see Chapter 2). However, even in well-treated supplies, some deposits may form in small diameter pipes and at dead-ends, and animals may be present (see Chapter 6). Deposits may also originate from historically poor water treatment. Some investigational work will be required to ensure that extensive internal encrustations of iron mains are not present. Where these exist, there is the risk that the adoption of an aggressive cleaning method will aggravate the problem by dislodging the encrustations and allowing the iron surfaces to "bleed" corrosion products. In badly encrusted pipes, the use of nonaggressive foam swabs is likely to be ineffective and the swabs could become stuck or disintegrate to create blockage problems.

A general approach to targeting pipes to be cleaned requires analysis of available water-quality information and maintenance records, and integration with other maintenance activities within the distribution system. Monitoring of swater-quality changes in the network can be used to identify baseline conditions and infer where deposits are located. The following parameters have been employed for this purpose (Cossins et al., 2000; Rodgers, Pizzi & Friedman, 1998; Friedman et al., 1998):

- heterotrophic bacteria counts and total coliforms
- residual disinfectant concentrations
- consumer complaints
- turbidity
- dissolved oxygen
- iron, aluminium and manganese concentrations.

The colour of filter-papers used to filter set volumes of water can indicate the internal condition of pipework. The method has been used to distinguish problems caused by corrosion, deposition of treatment chemicals and deposition of manganese (Evins, Leibeschuetz & Williams, 1990a).

Water-quality measurements may indicate the presence of deposits. The selection of a cleaning method (or indeed whether cleaning alone is appropriate) depends on the pipe material (easily identified if not known) and the nature of the deposits. The three nonaggressive methods described in this chapter are not suitable for the removal of:

- hard deposits such as calcium carbonate (downstream of water softening plants or in pipes conveying very "hard" waters);
- corrosion tubercles in iron pipes;
- adhesive deposits, such as those that are rich in manganese oxides.

Identifying the nature of the deposits in mains is difficult because they are relatively inaccessible. A number of water suppliers have used fibrescopes (fibre optic instruments), which allow visual inspection via mains tappings or hydrants under mains pressure (Carruthers & Evins, 1985). A more direct approach is the examination of pipe samples, exhumed deliberately for this purpose, or obtained opportunistically during repairs and system modifications. Other techniques involve controlled flushing via hydrants and washouts to estimate the quantities and measure the composition of loose deposits and the populations of animals (Evins, Liebeschuetz & Williams, 1990b).

4.3.3 Planning mains-cleaning programmes

Pipe-cleaning programmes require careful planning to be effective and to prevent flow conditions that may allow system contamination. For all three techniques, a basic principle is that water must enter the length of main being cleaned from a length of main that has been previously cleaned or is known to be clean. It is important to assess normal flow velocities and pressures, and the effects on these of the work being planned. An important hygiene requirement is to avoid low or negative pressures in adjacent parts of the network. A network model will help in this assessment and can be used to identify whether the planned operations will create flushing conditions in adjacent pipework. Planning will normally follow the eight steps listed below (Stephenson, 1989).

(1) Determine where cleaning is required (as described in Section 4.3.2) and which method to use (see Section 4.4 below).
(2) Prepare plans of the area(s) to be cleaned.
(3) Assess potential contamination hazards (low pressures, pipe environment, air valves, etc) and which preventative measures to adopt.
(4) Determine the timing of works and labour; determine plant and material requirements including those for good hygienic practice (see Chapter 5).
(5) Assess on-site traffic problems, access and condition of mains and valves.
(6) Review and, if necessary, modify, step 4.
(7) Brief operators, notify consumers, and arrange system modifications (e.g. tappings) if required.
(8) Monitor progress and effectiveness of the work.

The environmental impacts of an extensive pipe-cleaning programme should always be assessed beforehand. For example, the large volumes of water and deposits that are discharged will require careful disposal and dechlorination to avoid contamination of watercourses and land. It is prudent to inspect the site environment and address issues such options for discharge of dirty water, dechlorination, erosion, and potential scenarios for ingress and contamination.

Further to this, mitigation and protection measures should be considered, such as stormwater drain protection, temporary detention or off-site disposal.

Good consumer relations and information are critical to the success of a pipe-cleaning programme. Consumers, especially critical ones such as hospitals and other utilities, need to be informed of maintenance activities via a suitable communication strategy, which could include the following features:
- advance notification letters informing the community of forthcoming work; reasons and benefits to the water supply;
- shutdown notification (if required);
- handling of complaints and enquiries specific to the cleaning programme.

4.3.4 Monitoring effectiveness of mains cleaning

The parameters used to identify the parts of the network requiring cleaning should be measured after cleaning. Indicator organisms should be included, to verify that the working practices were hygienic (Ashbolt, Grabow & Snozzi, 2001). Existing operational and verification monitoring can be used to assess how the pipes have responded to cleaning in the long term (> 1 month). Data collection before and after cleaning is essential for understanding the benefits, costs and secondary impacts of the cleaning programme (Friedman et al., 1998).

4.4 NONAGGRESSIVE PIPE CLEANING METHODS

4.4.1 Introduction

The most commonly used cleaning methods for routine maintenance are flushing, air scouring and swabbing. Other, more abrasive, methods are available for cleaning pipes before the renovation of water mains by coating with spray-on protective linings such as cement mortar or epoxy resin, or before the insertion of pipe liners such as polyethylene. Examples are high pressure water jetting, power boring with metal flails, and abrasive pigging devices (AWWA, 2001). However when these abrasive methods are used to clean iron pipe surfaces they should always be followed by a lining method, otherwise corrosion will continue apace, causing extensive water discolouration and deterioration. The characteristics of each of these nonaggressive cleaning methods are described in the following sections and are summarized in Table 4.3.

Table 4.3. Characteristics of the nonaggressive pipe cleaning methods.

	Flushing	Air scouring	Swabbing
Pipe sizes	Up to 150 mm in high-pressure areas	Up to 200 mm	Normally up to 1000 mm
Plant and materials	Hoses for disposal of large water volumes	Air scouring rig and compressor	Swabs, swab locators
System modifications	Existing hydrants usually employed	Additional hydrants, valves and injection points may be needed	Insertion points on larger pipes
Comments	Of limited use in low-pressure areas, potential to create extensive disturbance that may not be removed via flushing hydrant	More effective than flushing and can be used in low-pressure areas	Blockages may occur if swab lost

Sources: WRc (1994), Stephenson (1989).

4.4.2 Flushing

Flushing involves the discharge of water from pipes, generally through hydrants and washouts, to generate velocities in the pipe capable of removing accumulated material and biofilms inside the pipe and attached to its walls. This is the simplest of the pipe-cleaning techniques. The velocity required to suspend and flush out the deposits depends on particle size and specific gravity. Although most small animals are of low specific gravity (about 1), inorganic deposits may have a specific gravity of up to 3. Table 4.4 provides the volumetric flow rates required to transport loose particles of 0.2 mm diameter. Below this diameter, the minimum flow rate required falls quickly with particle size. Above this diameter, the effect of flushing diminishes rapidly.

Table 4.4. Flow rate required to suspend and transport solids of 0.2 mm particle size in water mains.

Pipe diameter (mm)	Flow rate (l/s) for specific gravity 1.5	Flow rate (l/s) for specific gravity 3.0
50	1.5	2.7
75	3.8	7.2
100	7.6	15.0
150	20.0	41.0
200	42.0	83.0

Source: Stephenson (1989).

Many water suppliers have a long history of implementing flushing programmes in one form or another, and to varying extents within the distribution system. Flushing may be used routinely to expel contaminants or in response to consumer complaints. These latter unplanned operations often involve opening hydrants in an area and leaving them open until certain water quality objectives are met (e.g. reduction or elimination of discolouration of water, or decreased turbidity of water). Flushing velocities are not necessarily maximized and the water used to flush a particular pipe may not have originated from clean or preflushed pipework.

For planned maintenance it is important to adopt a systematic approach based on unidirectional flushing. This means working to ensure that water enters from a previously cleaned main and water approaches the discharge point from one direction only. A particular section of pipe is isolated, typically by closing valves. The hydrants are then opened in a sequential manner, with the aim of increasing the velocity of water flowing through the pipe, thereby suspending sediments and flushing them out. In calculating flushing times it is important to remove at least twice the nominal volume of each main, because the suspended particulate matter moves more slowly than the water.

Advantages of flushing:
- simple to perform because it requires only 1 or 2 persons;
- relatively inexpensive to carry out in comparison with other cleaning techniques.

Disadvantages of flushing:
- uses a lot of water;
- limited effectiveness unless high flow velocities are achieved;
- unlikely to remove all the biofilm from the pipe;
- not suitable for larger diameter mains because it is usually not practicable to achieve the desired flushing velocity.

4.4.3 Swabbing

The swabbing process involves driving a cylindrical foam sponge (known as a swab) through pipes using water pressure. The swab has a diameter approximately 25% greater than the pipe it is being forced through. Various grades of swab are available, depending on the particular manufacturer's specifications. Typically, they come in three grades: soft, hard and scouring (WRc, 1994).

In practice, swabbing will be effective when the velocity of the water in the pipe is between 0.8 and 1.5 m/s. If the swab travels too fast it will remove less material and will suffer from wear and tear. To prevent the swab from tumbling, the ratio of length to diameter should be 2 for small diameters (< 100 mm) and 1.5 for larger diameters.

Swabbing will remove soft deposits but not the hard scales or corrosion products that may be present. It is usual to send between three and six swabs through a pipe to achieve adequate cleaning.

Swabs are normally inserted into pipes using existing fixtures such as hydrants, or insertion points such as swept-tees (T-branched connections, with the middle branch sweeping in at a shallow angle) specifically installed for this purpose. The insertion method will depend on the local engineering practices. However, all methods involve gaining access to the pipe interior and inserting a swab that will be in contact with both drinking-water and surfaces that are exposed to drinking-water. It is therefore essential that staff apply the same working practices and disinfection procedures as described in Chapter 5 for all equipment and materials (e.g. swabs) used in swabbing operations.

Advantages of swabbing:
- superior to flushing and air scouring in terms of removing sediments and biofilm from the pipe wall;
- has the potential to remove almost all biomass and sediment;
- uses less water than flushing;
- no diameter limitations because foam swabs can be manufactured for practically all pipe sizes;
- swabs can be manufactured with abrasive surfaces to assist in removing harder deposits from the pipe wall (but see comments above concerning corroded and tuberculated iron mains).

Disadvantages of swabbing:
- consumers may have to be isolated from supply during the cleaning operation;
- swabs may break up in the pipe, particularly in pipes with a high degree of internal corrosion or encrustations;
- more expensive than flushing;
- problems with collecting and disposing of contaminants — swabbing can produce a large amount of discoloured water that requires careful environmental planning for its disposal;
- swabs may become stuck in any unforeseen bore restriction, such as inserted length of smaller diameter pipe or tuberculated section;
- requires suitable points for insertion of swabs;
- swabs and any other materials or equipment used in the insertion process must be disinfected.

4.4.4 Air scouring

Air scouring involves the controlled injection of filtered, compressed air into pipes, usually via a hydrant (Stephenson, 1989). Given a continuous supply of water and air in the right proportions, discrete "slugs" of water are formed in the main and driven along by the compressed air at high velocity. There is no need to turn the water or air on and off to achieve this effect. This is illustrated in Figure 4.1. The high velocity slugs tend to lift up silt and sediment from the base of the pipe. Air-scouring companies do not claim that the process removes much, if any, biofilm from the walls of the pipe. Achieving the right conditions whereby high velocity 'slugs' are propelled through the pipework is a skilled task, and normally undertaken by a specialist team. Alternate slugs of air and water, along with loose sediments, are ejected from the hydrant (or other fixture) at the end of the pipe being cleaned. It is very important to get all the compressed air out of the pipe before it is returned to service, to avoid unstable flows and cloudy water.

The fact that pipeline fixtures will be used as air injection points dictates that the same hygienic working practices will be required as described above for swabbing. The additional complication is that ambient air is normally injected after being pressurized in an air compressor, which will almost certainly release oil into the air stream. Therefore, the compressed air should be passed through an air cooler and suitable filters to ensure removal of both oil droplets and oil vapours. The nature of the ambient air and its potential to contaminate the pipework should also be considered: for example, the proximity of a cooling tower generating aerosols could be considered potentially hazardous if the aerosols contain chemicals or microorganisms.

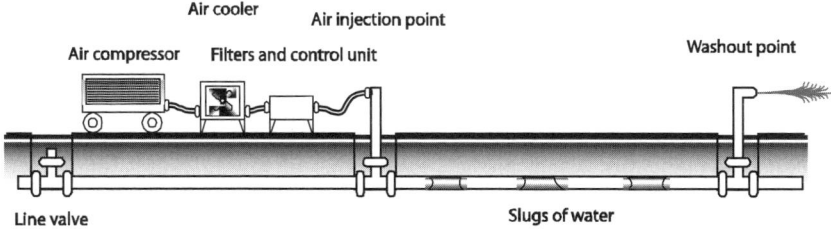

Figure 4.1. Achieving slug flow during air scouring.

Advantages of air scouring:
- about 40% less water is used during air-scouring than during swabbing or flushing;
- removes more deposits from pipes than flushing;
- the likelihood of a pipe break is very low as air pressure is kept below the static operating pressure of the pipe.

Disadvantages of air scouring:
- only effective in pipes with a diameter of less than 200 mm (also reported to lose its effectiveness in very small diameter pipes);
- not as effective as swabbing for removing biofilms;
- operators must be skilled, to ensure that the correct proportions of air and water are used;
- as with swabbing, consumers need to be isolated from the water supply during air scouring to ensure that discoloured water does not enter the house service pipes;
- precautions must be taken to prevent air contaminated with pathogens and chemicals (such as compressor oil) entering the pipework.

4.5 SUMMARY

Structural deficiencies in tanks, reservoirs, valves, fittings and pipework may offer direct routes for the contamination of water supplies with pathogens. This will depend on the environment surrounding the different components of the distribution system and the water pressure. Emergencies will generate low pressures in most conventional distribution systems.

Most tanks, reservoirs and fittings are accessible for inspection and planned maintenance. They should be prioritized according to sanitary risks, and surveyed and maintained in accordance with those risks. The survey and maintenance of service reservoirs is especially important because of the large populations served by these structures and the absence of internal water pressure at potential contamination points.

There are sound hygienic reasons for maintaining the internal cleanliness of pipework. Although there are no reports of health effects directly attributed to deposits in pipes, they do provide conditions for proliferation of microorganisms and animals. This may make the water unpalatable and make it difficult to identify contamination of hygienic significance by routine monitoring. The deposits also hinder the maintenance of a disinfectant residual, especially in the smaller diameter pipes which are at greatest risk of low pressures and hence contamination.

Pipe cleaning programmes can be used to maintain the internal cleanliness of a network. They require careful planning to be effective and to prevent flow conditions that may allow system contamination. It is important to assess normal flow velocities and pressures, and the effects on these of the work being planned. A network hydraulic model will help in this assessment. An important hygienic requirement is to avoid low or negative pressures in, and adjacent to, those parts of the network being cleaned. When using swabs or injected air to clean pipework, the materials and fixtures are potential sources of contamination and therefore the hygienic practices described in Chapter 5 should be followed.

4.6 REFERENCES

Ashbolt NJ, Grabow WOK, Snozzi M (2001). Indicators of microbial water quality. In: Fewtrell L, Bartram J, eds. *Water quality: guidelines, standards and health: risk assessment and management for water related infectious diseases.* IWA Publishing, London, UK.

AWWA (2001). *Rehabilitation of water mains*, 2nd ed. American Water Works Association, USA.

AWWARF (2001). *Pathogen intrusion into the distribution system.* American Water Works Association Research Foundation, Denver, USA.

Carruthers FB, Evins C (1985). *Fibre optic instruments for the internal inspection of water mains. A source document for the water mains rehabilitation manual.* Water Research Centre, Swindon, UK.

Cossins F et al. (2000) The Cincinnati water works' unidirectional flushing programme results and alternative approaches for full-scale implementation. In *American Water Works Association Conference Proceedings*, ISBN: 1583210733.

Evins C et al. (1989). *Planning the rehabilitation of water distribution systems. Principal document of the water mains rehabilitation manual.* Water Research Centre, Swindon, UK.

Evins C, Liebeschuetz J, Williams SM (1990a). *Aesthetic water quality problems in distribution systems. A source document for the water mains rehabilitation manual.* Water Research Centre, Swindon, UK, Appendix H.

Evins C, Liebeschuetz J, Williams SM (1990b). *Aesthetic water quality problems in distribution systems. A source document for the water mains rehabilitation manual.* Water Research Centre, Swindon, UK, Chapter 2.

Friedman M et al. (1998). Developing and implementing a distribution system flushing programme. *American Water Works Association Conference Proceedings*, 16.

Herz RK (1998). Exploring rehabilitation needs and strategies for water distribution systems. *Journal of Water Supply: Research and Technology — Aqua*, 47(6):275–283.

Lei J, Sægrov S (1998). Statistical approach for describing failures and lifetimes of water mains. *Water Science and Technology*, 38(6):209-217.

Rodgers ML, Pizzi NG, Friedman M (1998). Distribution flushing to improve corrosion control and water quality. *American Water Works Association Conference Proceedings*, 9.

Stephenson G (1989). *Removing loose deposits from water mains: operational guidelines. Source document for the water mains rehabilitation manual.* Water Research Centre, Swindon, UK.

Tarbet NK, Thomas BJ, Brown JA (1993). *Service reservoirs operation, repair and maintenance.* Report No. 1409 UM, Water Research Centre, Swindon, UK.

Taylor JW, Gary GW Jr, Greenberg HB (1981). Norwalk-related viral gastroenteritis due to contaminated drinking water. *American Journal of Epidemiology*, 114:584–592.

Walski TM (1994). Valves and distribution system reliability. *Proceedings of American Water Works Association Annual Conference*, New York, 1994. American Water Works Association, USA, 599–613.

WRc (1994). *Water mains cleaning handbook.* Water Research Centre, Swindon, UK.

5
Precautions during construction and repairs

Richard Ainsworth and David Holt

5.1 INTRODUCTION

Engineering work on distribution systems presents risks of widespread contamination of water supplies. The risks depend on factors such as the degree of pollution at the construction or repair site, the method of construction or repair, the ability to contain potential contamination by valving and, most importantly, the cleanliness of personnel, their working practices and the materials employed. The following activities may present risks of contamination with pathogenic microorganisms:
- construction of new pipework or the abandonment of existing pipework;
- renovation work using either structural or nonstructural linings, such as polyethylene slipliners or spray-on coatings;

© 2004 World Health Organization. *Safe Piped Water: Managing Microbial Water Quality in Piped Distribution Systems*. Edited by Richard Ainsworth. ISBN: 1 84339 039 6. Published by IWA Publishing, London, UK.

- repairs, either emergency or planned, that involve pressure loss or breaking into the inside of a pipe;
- reconnecting a water main after it has been taken out of service for an extended period.

Emergency repairs present the greatest risks — locating valves, dealing with consumers and traffic, the presence of adjacent services and the need to restore an essential supply all create difficulties when the location and timing are unplanned. Minimizing the risks arising from both emergency and planned engineering work depends on:
- having documented protocols;
- adopting general precautionary working practices;
- using health criteria to select personnel;
- implementing effective procedures for cleaning and disinfection;
- assessing the risks and monitoring the effects of both planned and emergency engineering work.

This chapter addresses each of these topics, with an emphasis on recent assessments of the efficacy of traditional approaches to cleaning and disinfecting water mains after construction, planned maintenance and emergency repairs. Box 5.1 provides an example of a disease outbreak associated with a broken water main.

Box 5.1. An outbreak of jaundice associated with a broken water main.

In January 1990, the staff at Rairangpur Hospital in Orisa, India noticed a sharp increase in the number of patients admitted because of jaundice. A community survey was conducted to identify further cases. About a fifth of the population were contacted and 127 cases of jaundice were identified as occurring in December or January, giving an estimated size of the outbreak of 635 cases, with one death. Serological tests were negative for both hepatitis A and B, making this non-A, non-B hepatitis (presumably the outbreak was hepatitis E).

The city of Rairangpur has 15 wards, of which 9 had an intermittent piped water supply and 6 had to rely on hand pumps and dug wells. The town had no sewerage system and open-air defecation was the general practice. The distribution of cases of jaundice was strongly correlated with water source. People who used the piped supply were nine times more likely to have developed jaundice than people who used the dug wells.

On investigation, it was found that a main pipe had burst on December 1st, though this was promptly repaired. This pipe supplied water to the five wards with the highest attack rates. This example illustrates the importance of sanitary conditions in the vicinity of water mains undergoing repair and maintenance.
Source: Bora et al.(1993).

As for other aspects of water supply hygiene, it is important that procedures are developed for local circumstances and are incorporated in national codes of practice, and in training and instructions for waterworks staff. The national codes of practice should also be reviewed regularly in the light of local performance and international technical developments.

5.2 PRECAUTIONARY WORKING PRACTICES

Typical guidance concerning hygienic working practices usually includes general advice on prevention measures. The following advice has been abstracted from two sets of guidelines (Water UK, 1998; AWWA, 1999).

- When working with pipes and fittings on site, ensure that they are protected from contamination by storing off the ground, capping the ends of pipes and liners, and keeping fittings in wrappings until the time of use (see Box 5.2).
- Ensure that the open ends of pipes in trenches are plugged and watertight when not being worked on or when there is a risk of the trench flooding.
- Excavate trenches to below the pipe level to provide a sump, and keep as dry as possible to prevent water entering a pipe or fitting.
- Ensure that sealing materials and lubricants are clean and certified as suitable for contact with potable water supplies.
- Protect unattended trenches and engineering sites from vandals and animals.
- If a part of the distribution system has been taken out of service for an extended period, treat it as a potentially contaminated new installation. Apply the flushing, disinfection and microbiological sampling procedures that are normally applied to new installations (see below).
- If a part of the distribution system is to be abandoned, ensure that all boundaries with the live system are effectively closed with especially secure and marked valves, or are capped. Create boundaries to minimize dead legs on the live system and ensure that the location of the abandoned system is recorded for future reference.
- When planning new installations and renovation works, make sure that the plans include valves, injection and washout points to facilitate effective cleaning and disinfection of the pipework.
- As far as is practicable, if general purpose or specialized vehicles are used for water supply construction and repair duties, do not use those vehicles for other duties where contamination may be prevalent (e.g. sewerage work).

- Clearly mark equipment and materials used in contact with water supplies as intended for this purpose and protect them from direct contamination with sewage or sewage sludge.

Box 5.2. A foxy tale.

A few months after moving into their homes, residents of a new housing estate started to complain of pieces of fur and other particles appearing in their tap water. The estate was supplied with water through a 15 cm diameter main that fed into a circular main round the estate. The diameter of the pipe tapered down to 10 cm.

The cause of the particulate material was traced to a dead fox. The fox had apparently climbed into the system during construction and, when the pipe had been charged, had become stuck at the taper. Because the estate was supplied by a loop system, the flow of water to consumers' taps was not interrupted. As the fox decayed it started to break up and at this point small pieces of rotting flesh appeared in consumers' tap water.

Microbiological analysis showed heavy contamination of the system with coliforms and *Escherichia coli*. Residents of the estate had to be evacuated while the supply and the domestic plumbing systems were thoroughly cleaned.

This example illustrates the importance of ensuring that mains pipes are kept capped at all times when they are not being directly supervised.

Source: Anonymous.

5.3 PERSONNEL

Known carriers of potentially waterborne communicable diseases should not come into contact with the distribution system of potable water supplies. The local circumstances and environment will dictate which diseases pose the greatest threats and how best to employ and monitor personnel to minimize such risks. However, certain guidance concerning good practice is universally applicable, as described below.

- Water supply activities that pose a potential contamination risk should be defined and given a clear descriptive name. For example, in the United Kingdom, such activities are referred to as "restricted operations" and this terminology is used below.
- Employees and contractors involved in restricted operations should be trained in the hygienic implications of their work and basic hygienic practices. This training should include details of the personal symptoms that indicate a potential waterborne disease. All staff (employees and contractors) should be encouraged to report such symptoms without prejudice to their employment prospects.

- Employers should provide adequate toilet and washing facilities to maintain personal hygiene. Wastes from portable or temporary arrangements should be disposed of without risk to water supplies or the environment.
- A medical officer should review the suitability of individuals for restricted operations at regular intervals. This may involve the use of questionnaires.

5.4 CLEANING AND DISINFECTION PROCEDURES

Before putting into service a new, repaired, rehabilitated or modified water main carrying potable water, the main must first be cleaned, disinfected, flushed and sampled to ensure that it is free from contamination. Each stage is important, but the emergence of knowledge concerning the resistance of *Cryptosporidium* oocysts to high concentrations of disinfectants such as aqueous chlorine (WRc, 1988) has placed extra emphasis on the removal of all solid matter from the interior of pipes and fittings before reconnection. Furthermore, deposits left in mains may shield pathogens from the disinfectant and allow them to remain undetected during subsequent microbiological sampling. A main may appear satisfactory, but deposits may then be disturbed and contaminate the conveyed water. Chemical disinfection, even in relatively high doses, should never be considered a catch-all stage for ensuring hygienic conditions in a new or repaired distribution system; physical removal of all introduced deposits is a critical control stage. Some water suppliers recognize this by requiring that all new mains incorporate swab (usually polyurethane foam) insertion and removal points, to allow future maintenance and to swab the newly laid main before flushing and disinfection.

The presence of deposits previously formed in a main that is being repaired obviously creates problems when assessing whether contamination has occurred or whether cleaning has been effective. However, introduced material is likely to be less adhesive than indigenous deposits, and vigorous flushing and swabbing should be effective if well controlled.

5.4.1 Typical cleaning and disinfection procedures

Guidance concerning cleaning and disinfection procedures is an important component of water safety plans, as described in Chapter 7. The guidance typically differentiates between practices for new constructions and repairs. Tables 5.1 and 5.2 list advice contained in two readily available sets of guidelines (Water UK, 1998 and WAA, 1988; AWWA, 1999); they are given here for illustration.

Table 5.1. Recommended practice for new mains and inserted liners.

	Recommended practice[a]		Recommended practice[b]
1	Remove introduced material by flushing or other means (i.e. swabbing)	1	Flush main until clear.
2	Disinfect at initial free chlorine concentration of 25 mg/l for 24 hours. With chlorinated water: • achieve a residual of 10 mg/l if using continuous feed • dose at 100 mg/l of free chlorine for 3 hours if using slug feed.	2	Disinfect at initial free chlorine concentration of 20 mg/l for 16 hours or equivalent.
3	Flush until chlorine concentrations are equivalent to normal mains feed	3	Flush out disinfectant solution.
		4	Recharge with mains water for further 24 hours.
4	Take two consecutive sets of samples (at least 24 hours apart) along the main for bacteriological analysis.	5	Take samples along the main for bacteriological analysis.
5	Bring into service if samples are free of coliforms.	6	Bring into service if samples are free of coliforms, and if main contents are of acceptable appearance and free of taste and odour (minimum criteria).

Source: a, AWWA (1999); b, Water UK (1998) & WAA (1988).

Table 5.2. Recommended practice for repairs to mains.

	Recommended practice[a]		Recommended practice[b]
			Repair on live main without loss of pressure and without cutting (i.e. using repair clamp)
		1	Disinfect fracture area and fitting with solution containing 1000 mg/l of free chlorine.
		2	Return to service.
	Repair on wholly or partially dewatered mains		*Repair on cut main*
1	Disinfect cut area and fittings with 10 000 mg/l hypochlorite solution.	1	Disinfect cut area and fittings with solution containing 1000 mg/l of free chlorine.
2	Flush until no discolouration. If possible flush towards the work location from both directions.	2	Flush main section.
3	Where practical, isolate section of main and service connections, and chlorinate as for new mains (dose may be increased to 300 mg/l for 15 minutes), then flush to remove chlorine and any discolouration.	3	If possibility of internal contamination from vicinity of repair, charge main with chlorine solution (e.g. concentration of 20 mg/l for 2 hours or 50 mg/l for 30 minutes), then flush out.
4	Sample for bacteriological contamination to provide record of efficacy. Continue until two consecutive sets are negative.	4	Sample for bacteriological contamination.
5	Return to service	5	Return to service unless the potential internal contamination was from a sewer or similar high risk source. If so obtain prior written clearance (from operations scientist or similar).

Source: a, AWWA (1999); b, Water UK (1998) & WAA (1988).

In the case of mains undergoing renovation with spray-on linings (or similar) guidance is usually similar to that for a repair with potential internal contamination. However, additional flushing and testing is likely to be required to avoid unacceptable levels of chemical contaminants leaching from such linings.

5.4.2 Methods for dosing chlorine into the mains

Gaseous chlorine is not a practical option for field disinfection applications because it poses a safety risk for utility staff, contractors and the public. Calcium hypochlorite (as granules or tablets) and sodium hypochlorite solution are the normal chemicals of choice for this situation.

Quantities of calcium hypochlorite may be deposited in the main at regular intervals during construction or during a repair. The recommended quantities, spatial distribution and maximum filling velocity for the inlet water are a function of pipe internal diameter. Detailed guidelines are available (AWWA, 1999). The objective is to achieve an initial dose of 25 mg/l of free chlorine and to have a detectable chlorine residual after 24 hours. Some codes restrict the use of calcium hypochlorite to, for example, short lengths or emergency repairs to burst mains. Important limitations are:
- the need to keep the main clean and dry in a new construction to prevent premature dissolution;
- the presence of the solid hypochlorite, which precludes any preliminary flushing;
- the tendency of the dissolution process to concentrate the dense hypochlorite solution at the bottom of the pipe.

Sodium hypochlorite solution can be prepared in concentrated form and then dosed proportionally to flow into the main, or dosed in batch form if a tank is available. These solutions are corrosive and should be treated with caution. The flow can then be stopped when the main is full, or it can be continuously fed through the main to waste. The American Water Works Association standard (AWWA, 1999), which provides detailed guidance, refers to the former as the "slug method" and to the latter as the "continuous method". The slug method creates less volume of chlorinated water to be disposed of and uses less chemical; the continuous method can provide a uniform concentration of chlorine along the length of main. Recommended concentrations and contact times are summarized in Table 5.1.

Detailed practical information on the manufacture of chlorine solutions, chlorine measurement, destruction of chlorine residues in wastewater and flushing volumes is available (e.g. AWWA, 1999).

5.4.3 Practical problems

New construction work and renovation should present few problems because there is time available to plan carefully and to forewarn consumers. Also, the interior of the pipework is new or resurfaced and has a smooth bore, free of encrustation and corrosion. This assists in cleaning the pipe and should reduce chlorine consumption during the disinfection stage. However, some linings may themselves exert a chlorine demand and make it difficult to achieve target chlorine residuals. This has been observed during investigations of cement mortar linings applied in-situ (Rayner, Olliffe & Kings, 1993).

The majority of problems occur when making emergency repairs. The ability to quickly locate valves, stopcocks and washout points relies on good local knowledge or accessible records. Consumers may need to be warned and may have to move out of the buildings involved. Finding a convenient injection and washout point may require the isolation of a long length of main, especially in a rural area. Furthermore, the existing pipework may contain deposits and encrustation that consume the disinfectant.

These practical concerns have lead to a reappraisal of the effectiveness of the traditional cleaning and disinfection practices in recent years, as outlined in the next section.

5.4.4 Effectiveness of guidance for field disinfection

An underground pipe rig and field trials have been used to identify the performance of various disinfection practices and cleaning practices used in the UK (WRc, 1994). In a series of experiments, the dispersion of chlorine in small diameter mains (< 150 mm) was first investigated. The results demonstrated the poor and nonuniform dispersion of disinfectant that occurs when either solid or dissolved hypochlorite is introduced at one end of a pipe and then distributed by the incoming water used to charge the main. Dosing calcium hypochlorite tablets at the spacing recommended by the manufacturers reduced the nonuniformity of the distribution, but target doses were not achieved at some locations. As would be expected, dosing sodium hypochlorite solution into water being used to charge the main was most effective.

In the same investigation, the effects of various combinations of chlorine concentrations and contact times (with and without prior swabbing) were measured. The method of measurement was unusual in that the biofilm on a standardized area of the pipe interior was sampled and the bacteria enumerated using a heterotrophic plate count technique. Other investigations have relied on sampling the conveyed water. The experiments used either exhumed or in situ cast-iron pipes, which were tuberculated with corrosion products and contained established biofilms. The results were variable because of variation in the size of the bacterial colonies on the pipe surfaces. However, chlorine consumption was found to be more a function of the indigenous deposits than of the introduced deposits in pipes of this condition. Conventional doses and contact times reduced general bacterial numbers on the surfaces by 65–98%, although preswabbing appeared to have no beneficial effect in such circumstances. These results indicate that normal doses of chlorine are able to affect the bacterial populations on surfaces and hence provide some safeguard in case of certain pathogens entering pipes during construction and repair (although the disinfectant is ineffective against pathogens such as viruses and the oocysts of protozoa). The results also indicate the benefits of routine maintenance activities intended to keep the system free of deposits and biofilms.

Similar investigations have been undertaken to identify the performance of various disinfection and cleaning practices used in the USA (AWWARF, 1998). These investigations measured bacterial numbers in water that had been flushed through pipe rigs containing new pipes and old used pipes. In some cases, water flushed from the vicinity of mains breaks was used. The purpose was to identify bacterial numbers that occur on pipe surfaces and to study the disinfection kinetics within the water itself. The results were as follows.

- None of the water mains tested was found to have detectable total coliforms or acid-fast bacteria but all mains (including new ones) had high heterotrophic bacteria counts.
- Heterotrophic bacteria counts in used mains were variable, but were comparable to levels in new mains. Tuberculated used mains had higher counts than smooth bore used mains.
- All mains (including new ones) exhibited a significant chlorine demand.
- In all cases, regardless of material, diameter or age of pipe, using an initial chlorine residual of 25 mg/l and a contact time of 24 hours resulted in a four-log inactivation of heterotrophic bacteria. This, of course, applied to the flushed organisms, not those remaining on the pipe surfaces.

The results of the American Water Works Association Research Foundation (AWWARF) study confirmed that the recommended procedures are a conservative approach to disinfecting conventional indicator and heterotrophic microorganisms. The authors did, however, point out that disinfectant-resistant pathogens such as *Giardia* and *Cryptosporidium* had not been investigated in the same way and that this is an outstanding research requirement.

5.5 RISK ASSESSMENT AND MONITORING

The decision on when to commission a newly constructed or repaired water main depends on the risk of contamination, the risk that cleaning and disinfection will be ineffective, and the added security that can be provided by satisfactory results arising from bacteriological sampling. With repairs, these risks need to be balanced against the practicalities associated with interruptions to supply.

When undertaking new constructions, renovation work and planned repairs it is normal to have sufficient time available to follow all the recommended procedures for dealing with materials, excavations, physical cleaning and long-duration disinfection. In such cases, risks are already low and added security is provided by sampling the main at regular intervals along its length and by testing for coliform organisms (at the very least). The AWWA standard recommends that two consecutive sets of acceptable samples, taken at least 24 hours apart, should be obtained before recommissioning (AWWA, 1999). The Water UK guidelines recommend that new mains be charged with mains water for 24 hours, sampled at appropriate points and analysed for residual chlorine, coliforms, turbidity, taste, odour and appearance (Water UK, 1998). Mains that fail such tests will obviously require investigation and should be reflushed (or recleaned by some other means such as swabbing), rechlorinated and sampled until acceptable results are obtained, before commissioning the main.

Emergency repairs create obvious difficulties in comparison with planned work. Water suppliers are confronted with balancing the risks of contamination with the risks of poor sanitary conditions occurring in the absence of a mains supply. Table 5.2 summarizes the advice provided by two national codes. The important requirement is good site practice and information. If a break causes pressure loss and is near a leaking sewer or contaminated ground, then extreme caution should be exercised before recommissioning; a larger area may need to be cleaned. In such cases, the decision should be made by a suitably qualified employee of the water supplier.

Bacteriological sampling after emergency repairs may not inform the decision to return the affected pipe to service because of the delay in obtaining microbiological results. However, these samples are still important. They provide baseline data in the event of a problem developing subsequently; they also provide a record of the effectiveness of an organisation's working practices; indeed they may reveal differences in the performance of different repair crews. These data should be regularly reviewed to identify areas for improvement.

Box 5.3 (below) describes an outbreak of giardiasis associated with work on a water main.

5.6 SMALL COMMUNITY-MANAGED SYSTEMS

It is important to follow hygienic working practices during construction of community-managed piped supplies; also, the supply should be properly disinfected before commissioning. Training in good hygiene practices for repair work is essential for operators and managers of such supplies.

> **Box 5.3.** An outbreak of giardiasis associated with work on a water main.
>
> An outbreak of giardiasis affected residents of Bristol, England during the summer of 1985. There were 108 laboratory confirmed cases. Most of the cases were resident in an area supplied by a single reservoir and became ill during the middle two weeks of July. Epidemiological investigations showed a very strong association between illness and consumption of unboiled tap water in the affected area during the first week of July. Data from water samples taken from the reservoir and the distribution of cases suggested that contamination occurred after water had left the reservoir.
>
> Although the exact cause of failure was not identified, the outbreak coincided with work on the implicated mains. The main had been opened on two separate occasions for a few hours. It was suggested that either this had allowed access to infected water or had allowed backflow into the mains during the pressure drop.
>
> This outbreak demonstrates the dangers associated with work on the distribution system. The potential risks to public health should be considered before any work on the distribution system.
>
> Source: Jephcott, Begg & Baker (1986).

Community operators and managers need to have a good understanding of where the distribution system is laid, and a diagram of the system that shows pipe location in relation to easily recognized landmarks. This is particularly important in older systems where changes in community operator or management committee may have occurred. It may be necessary for an external agency (such as a surveillance body) to ensure that this knowledge is maintained, through periodic visits.

Training of community operators should include hygienic working practices, and guidance material should be provided to the operator as a reference. This material should be simple and attractive, and should maximize the use of pictures (even in literate communities).

Simple guidance should be provided to communities regarding good hygiene during work carried out on pipes, based on the practices outlined above. These may need modification to remove those that are obviously not applicable (e.g. the use of specialized vehicles) and to include additional guidance that is appropriate.

Within small, community-managed systems, medical checks on personnel working on pipelines are often not feasible. It must therefore be emphasized to community operators and managers that people who are currently suffering from diarrhoea or who have recently had diarrhoea should not undertake work on distribution systems.

5.7 SUMMARY

The hygienic safety of repaired or constructed pipework is dependent on good working practice and the removal of all debris and water that may have entered a pipe. Disinfection, although important, is not a panacea for contaminated pipework, especially as some pathogens may be resistant.

Recent investigations of published guidelines for the cleaning and disinfection of new and repaired water mains show these to be effective when followed carefully. However, existing deposits and encrustations in water mains may consume much of the disinfectant.

Chlorination using an externally prepared solution of hypochlorite to charge the whole main gives the best dispersion of disinfectant. Introducing hypochlorite tablets or a volume of hypochlorite solution followed by charging the main is a much less effective means of uniform dispersion.

The construction and renovation of mains provides an opportunity to incorporate valves, and injection and washout points for swabs or for flushing. These will facilitate immediate cleaning and disinfection of the pipework, and will be useful in the long-term maintenance of the system.

Good hygiene is equally vital during work on the distribution system in small, community-managed water supplies. Providing proper training and simple guidance material to support safe, hygienic working practices in such supplies is essential.

5.8 REFERENCES

AWWA (1999). *AWWA standard for disinfecting water mains. Revision of ANSI/AWWA C651-92*. American Water Works Association, Denver, USA.

AWWARF (1998). *Development of disinfection guidelines for the installation and replacement of water mains*. American Water Works Association Research Foundation, Denver, USA.

Bora D et al. (1993). Epidemiology of a jaundice outbreak in Rairangpur Town in Orisa. *Journal of Communicable Diseases*, 25:1–5.

Jephcott AE, Begg NT, Baker IA (1986). Outbreak of giardiasis associated with mains water in the United Kingdom. *Lancet*, 1:730–732.

Rayner H, Olliffe T, Kings KM (1993). *durability and environmental impact of cement mortar linings, second year report*. Report No. FR0369, Foundation for Water Research, Marlow, UK.

WAA (1988). *Operational guidelines for the protection of drinking water supplies*. Water Authorities Association (now Water UK), London.

WRc (1994). *Guidelines for field disinfection of water mains*. Report No. UC 2380. Water Research Centre, Swindon, UK.

WRc (1988). *The effect of free chlorine on the viability of* Cryptosporidium *spp oocysts*. Report No. 2023 PRU. Water Research Centre, Swindon, UK.

Water UK (1998). *Principles of water supply hygiene and technical guidance notes. Technical papers*. Water UK, London.

6
Small animals in drinking-water distribution systems

Colin Evins

6.1 INTRODUCTION

Invertebrate animals are naturally present in many water resources used as sources for the supply of drinking-water. Small numbers of adults or their larvae may pass through water-treatment works if the barriers to particulate matter are not completely effective. Their motility may also enable them to penetrate filters at the treatment works and vents on storage reservoirs.

Many of these animals can survive (and some may even reproduce) within the supply network by deriving their food from the microorganisms and organic matter in the water or (more commonly) present in deposits on pipe and tank surfaces. Populations of small animals are surprisingly widespread in treated-water distribution systems. Reports from most continents suggest that few, if any, water distribution systems are completely free of animals. However, the density and composition of animal populations vary widely, from heavy

© 2004 World Health Organization. *Safe Piped Water: Managing Microbial Water Quality in Piped Distribution Systems*. Edited by Richard Ainsworth. ISBN: 1 84339 039 6. Published by IWA Publishing, London, UK.

infestations of readily visible species that are objectionable to consumers, to sparse occurrences of microscopic species. In spite of their ubiquity, these animal populations have not been widely studied and their biology is not well understood.

In temperate countries, no population of pathogenic animals has been found, or would be expected to be found, in a distribution system. The presence of animals has largely been regarded by water suppliers as an 'aesthetic' problem, either directly or through their association with discoloured water. However, there have been suggestions that their presence may affect the microbiological quality of water.

In tropical and subtropical countries, certain species of aquatic animal can act as secondary hosts for parasites. For example, the small crustacean *Cyclops* is the intermediate host of *Dracunculus medinensis*, the guinea worm — the only parasite that is known to be transmitted solely by water consumption (WHO, 1996). However there is no evidence that guinea worm transmission occurs from treated-water piped supplies.

In all countries, the presence of living animals or animal debris will reduce the acceptability of a water supply. People may then change to alternative supplies that may be less safe. Thus, for reasons of public health, it is important to prevent the entry and proliferation of animals in water distribution networks.

This chapter discusses:
- the occurrence and significance of metazoan (many-celled) animals in treated drinking-water distribution systems;
- the limited information available on their relationship with the microbiological quality of water and health concerns;
- methods of controlling populations of animals in the supply network.

This chapter does not deal with animals infesting raw water pipelines.

6.2 OCCURRENCE OF ANIMALS IN DISTRIBUTION SYSTEMS

6.2.1 Extent

There are reports in the literature of animals in water distribution systems from North America, Europe, Africa, South Asia and East Asia, from the late 19th century (before the widespread introduction of filtration and disinfection) into the 21st century. For example, the animal populations of water distribution systems were studied in the United Kingdom in the 1960s and 1970s; about 50 systems were sampled, and animals were found in all of them, although the water suppliers and their consumers were often unaware of their presence. About 150 species of animal were identified (Smalls & Greaves,

1968), including a species that had not been recorded from natural waters since the 1920s, but had been found in several water distribution systems. A systematic survey in the 1990s of water distribution systems supplied by 36 treatment works in the Netherlands also found animals in all of them, although fewer taxa were identified (van Lieverloo, 1997). Water pipes evidently provide a favourable environment for a variety of small aquatic animals.

No systematic studies have followed the numbers of animals present in distribution systems over a long period. Ad hoc observations from water suppliers suggest that, where the efficacy of water treatment has improved, animal numbers have probably declined.

6.2.2 Sampling

The usual method of sampling animals in water pipes is to flush a standard volume of water from a hydrant at a controlled flow rate, and to capture particulate matter, including animals, in a fine-meshed sampling net. The catch is sorted in a trough with a through flow of water, the species identified and their number estimated. Results are often only semiquantitative, the number of individuals of a particular species in a sample being expressed as an order of magnitude (1–9, 10–99, 100–999 etc.) (Smalls & Greaves, 1968).

More elaborate methods have been proposed. Van Lieverloo (1997) used a device that split the flow from the hydrant, part being filtered through a 500 μm mesh, and part being passed through an additional 100 μm mesh. Smart (1989) used repeated flushing of the same hydrant, and extrapolated from the declining numbers found in successive samples from the same point to estimate the total population in the length of main being sampled. Because different species show a different propensity to be flushed from the pipe, it was necessary to make a separate extrapolation for each. However, such methods have not found widespread favour, partly because it is uncertain how representative samples are, and partly because the considerable effort involved in making the sampling and counting more quantitative is usually not thought to be worthwhile for making short-term operational decisions. Consequently, few data exist on the biomass of the various species or on the dynamics of the ecosystems in water mains.

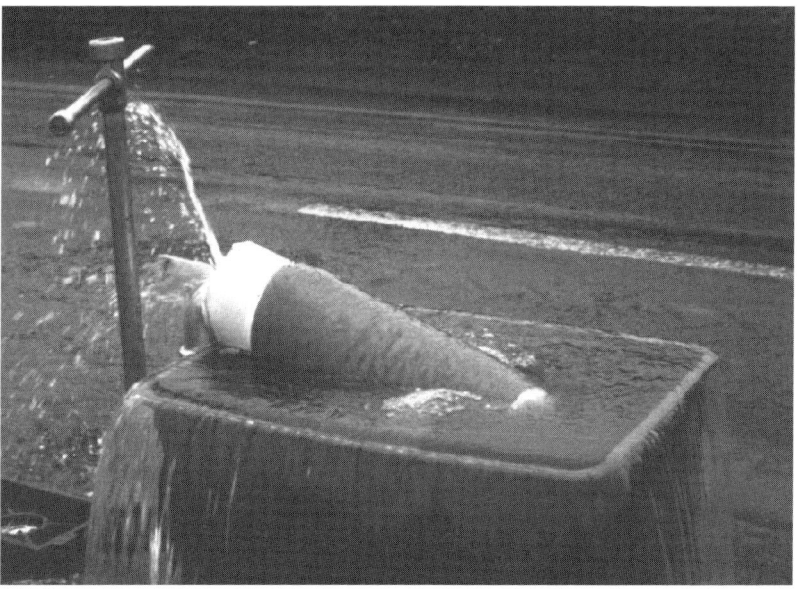

Plate 6.1. Sampling animals and loose deposits in a fine-meshed sampling net.

6.2.3 Ingress

Animals may be present in water distribution systems because:
- they enter the distribution system with the incoming water, having passed through treatment processes or having colonised parts of the treatment plant;
- they enter through defects in the integrity of the distribution system, such as badly screened service reservoirs;
- they form breeding populations within the distribution systems.

Animals that are aquatic for the whole or part of their life-cycle may gain initial entry to the system by penetration through treatment works. The animals that successfully penetrate treatment processes are largely benthic species (Evins & Greaves, 1979) — that is, species that live on the bottoms or margins of water bodies. Where water from upland reservoirs of good microbiological quality with a low content of suspended solids receives only limited treatment, planktonic species may enter the distribution system in appreciable numbers. However, they do not usually thrive there. Some benthic species have also been found to colonise filter beds and other parts of treatment works, and this has been shown to influence the numbers and species in the treated water leaving the works. The relative importance of this mechanism is unclear, but the species found in each situation suggest that it in most cases it is probably less important than the direct passage of animals with the water being treated.

Service reservoirs may be a point of entry for species that are aerial for part of their life-cycle. For example, flying insects may enter through badly protected vents and overflows, and lay eggs at the water surface, which develop into aquatic larvae. Significant ingress of chironomid (gnat) larvae may take place in this way. Terrestrial species may enter as a result of inadequate care in laying mains or through cracks and poorly fitting access covers at service reservoirs; the resulting problems are transient and cease when the access point is blocked.

The ingress of small numbers of aquatic animals through treatment works and the establishment of breeding populations in the distribution system is responsible for by far the greatest number of individuals. The initial entry of a species may have been some time ago, when water treatment was less effective than it is now, or it may be the result of periodic treatment failures.

Although a large proportion of the species that penetrate treatment works are benthic, and all those that thrive in the mains are benthic, it is not necessarily the species that pass treatment in the greatest numbers that are most common in the mains. A survey (Evins & Greaves, 1979) of treatment works and their associated distribution systems showed that, for most species, it is success of reproduction within the main that determines the size of the population. Thus, the species that are common in the distribution system are not necessarily those that appear most frequently at consumers' taps (van Lieverloo, 1997). This is because the species that thrive in the pipework may resist dislodgement and suspension in the conveyed water, whereas those that are present in the incoming supply may pass directly to consumers' taps.

Only animals that are aquatic for the whole of their life-cycle can colonise the distribution system and form breeding populations there. This excludes most insect larvae. Nevertheless, larvae of many species of chironomid may be present in the distribution system in appreciable numbers. Larvae are often present in large numbers in rivers and reservoirs, and may penetrate treatment works. These insects may colonise filter beds, they may also lay eggs in open tanks in treatment works or in badly protected service reservoirs.

However, several species of chironomid are parthenogenetic (females are able to reproduce without males), and have eggs that begin to develop within the pupa. In at least one species, *Paratanytarsus grimmii*, and possibly others, if emergence of the (normally aerial) imago is prevented (e.g. by lack of access to air) viable eggs are released from the pupa. Thus, successful reproduction is possible within the confines of water mains, and these insects have been particularly troublesome in water distribution systems in Europe and North America. (Krüger, 1941; Williams, 1974; Berg, 1995).

6.2.4 Population size

For some species, numbers depend on ingress from outside the distribution system; however, for most species, there are breeding populations within the distribution system that interact to form an ecosystem. The size of these populations depends on intrinsic characteristics, such as their adaptability to conditions in a water pipe, their reproductive potential and external factors, such as temperature and (most importantly) food supply. The majority of the species that thrive in water mains feed in their natural habitats on particulate organic matter or plant material. For example, the chydorids, which are often the most numerous group, feed by filtering small particles from water close to solid surfaces. One of the most successful of the larger colonizers of water mains, *Asellus aquaticus*, is a detritivore (an organism that feeds on nonliving organic matter) and is a fairly indiscriminate feeder. The faeces of *Asellus* taken from iron water mains contain about 70% by weight of iron oxides (Water Research Association, United Kingdom, unpublished data). Other species may graze more directly on surface biofilms.

Populations of these detritivores and grazers can flourish in the relative absence of pressure from carnivores. A number of small carnivorous species have been found, such as *Cyclops albidus*, which would feed on the smaller chydorids. However, larger carnivores are rare or absent. Fish are usually the 'top carnivores' in freshwater ecosystems, consuming invertebrates such as insect larvae, and are effectively absent from treated water distribution systems.

Thus, one may imagine that the food-chain in the water mains ecosystem is a relatively short one: most of the animal species present are at the same trophic level. They would be either competing directly for the same food supply of organic detritus and microorganisms, or using separate parts of it, divided for example by size and by whether or not they are attached to the substrate. Smart (1989) has studied the diversity of animals recolonising pipework following flushing. He found little pattern to the recolonisation in apparently similar situations, and concluded that there was a 'competitive lottery': the species which by chance arrived first being able to establish substantial populations.

Various observations and studies have shown a link between the type of water source, particularly its organic content, and the extent of animal populations in the water mains. Water from deep underground sources generally supports lower numbers of animals than water from surface sources, probably because water from underground has a low organic content. Increases in animals in the mains have been attributed to penetration of algae and to the introduction of treatment processes that are less effective at reducing the organic content of the water. Variations in the organic content of the water at one works have been linked to changes in the numbers of some groups of animals (Evins & Greaves, 1979), although these were unsophisticated studies. No known studies have quantified the interactions between the major elements of the system, namely the organic material entering the distribution system, the heterotrophic microorganisms in the pipework and the animals in the pipework.

It would be reasonable to suppose that the type of organic material is significant. Some particulate organic matter, such as algal cells and other plant material, may directly contribute to the food supply for filter feeders and detritivores. Increases in populations of *Asellus aquaticus* have been noted after high algal numbers in raw water, the introduction of water from surface sources and a change to treatment processes that were less effective at removing algae. Biodegradable dissolved organic material contributes to microbial growth (see Chapter 2) and thus to the food supply for animals, although the more refractory dissolved or colloidal organic material, such as the humic material prevalent in some upland waters, is likely to be less suitable.

As a generalization, the trophic interactions may be summarized as in Figure 6.1. The relationships involved have not been satisfactorily quantified. In particular, there is lack of information on the quantity of biofilm material necessary to support populations of grazing animals, and a corresponding lack of information on the effect of the grazing on the quantity and species composition of biofilms.

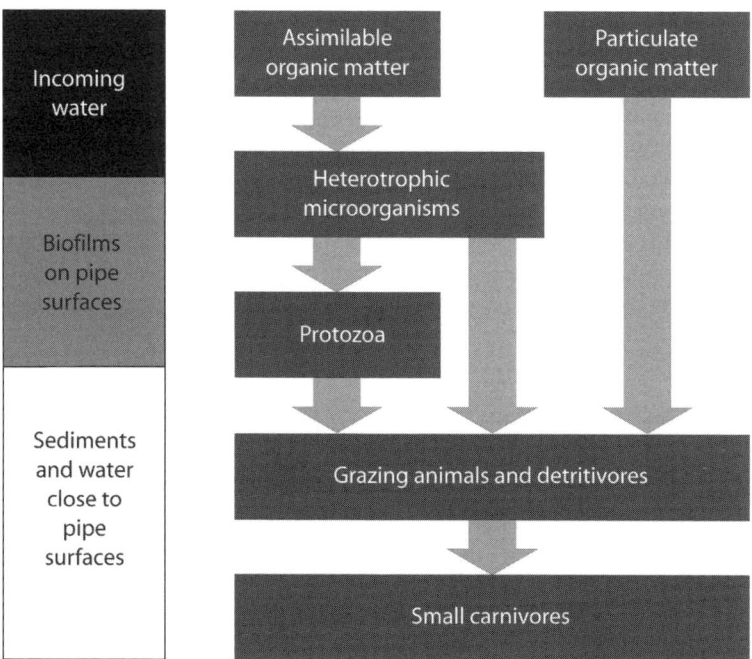

Figure 6.1. Generalized trophic interactions in water distribution systems.

Recommendations have been made to limit the potential for the growth of animal populations in water mains by limiting the amount of organic matter entering the distribution system (Evins, Liebeschuetz & Williams, 1990; van Lieverloo, 1997). The severity of infestations has declined in some countries in recent years; this may be related to improvements in the efficacy of water treatment not primarily introduced for this reason.

6.3 SIGNIFICANCE OF METAZOAN ANIMALS IN DRINKING-WATER DISTRIBUTION SYSTEMS

6.3.1 Aesthetic problems

The presence of animals has largely been regarded by water suppliers in temperate countries as an "aesthetic" problem. The few studies in distribution systems and the animal control activity by water suppliers have been concerned with the aesthetic aspects. The larger animals may be visible to the consumer and may be objectionable if they appear at the tap. Also, animals are associated with discoloured water problems as both cause and effect; the animals thrive at points of low flow, such as dead end mains and badly encrusted pipes, where sediments accumulate. Examination of samples of discoloured water has sometimes revealed that the particulate matter consists largely of fragments of animals, such as the cast carapaces of chydorids, which are stained with iron.

The decay of animals and their faeces may create the potential for taste and odour problems. Alternatively, the animals may have a beneficial effect — by feeding on particulate organic matter they limit the potential growth of microorganisms such as actinomycetes, which can cause taste and odour problems. Both these hypotheses are conjectural. In view of the much greater biomass of microorganisms than that of animals, and the known association between some of these microorganisms and odour problems, the beneficial effect seems more likely.

6.3.2 Metazoan parasites

In temperate countries, there is no evidence that any of the metazoan animals found in water distribution systems are directly harmful to human beings.

In tropical and subtropical countries, certain species of aquatic invertebrate animal act as intermediate hosts for parasites. The parasitic nematode *Dracunculus medinensis*, the guinea worm, presently occurs in sub-Saharan Africa only, but regions where it has been historically endemic also include North Africa, Middle East and the Indian subcontinent. It is transmitted solely by water consumption (WHO, 1996). *Cyclops* is its intermediate host: one larval stage develops within the crustacean, and human infection (dracunculiasis) results from ingesting water containing infected *Cyclops*. Further larval development and growth of the adult worm (up to 1 m in length) takes place in subcutaneous tissue. Juvenile worms are released: these cause a severe allergic reaction and ulceration, which often becomes infected by bacteria. The sufferer often uses water to cool the inflamed and infected areas, allowing the juvenile worms to return to water and infect new *Cyclops*. Thus, in areas where dracunculiasis is prevalent, raw water should be treated sufficiently well to remove *Cyclops*. However, there is no evidence that guinea worm transmission occurs from piped drinking-water supplies.

The five species of the parasitic flatworm *Schistosoma* that cause schistosomiasis (bilharziasis) have occurred in many countries in Central and South America, Africa, Asia Minor, South-East Asia and the Western Pacific (WHO, 1996). They have a complex aquatic life-cycle with aquatic snails as their intermediate hosts. Eggs released by human beings develop into miracidia, which are infective to snails, where they develop and release sporocysts. These in turn develop into cercariae, which are infective to human beings. Thus, in the tropical and subtropical regions where schistosomiasis is prevalent, the presence of snails in the distribution system could pose a hazard. If the snails are not already infected, it is possible they will become so if eggs or miracidia pass through treatment. Again, this is a theoretical risk and there is no evidence of piped distribution systems acting as a transmission route for this disease.

6.3.3 Effect of animals on occurrence of microorganisms in water mains

There have been suggestions that the presence of animals may have an effect on the microbial quality of water. Animals play a role in the biological equilibrium in the distribution system. The animals present in water mains occur predominantly in sediments or close to the pipe walls, and this is where microorganisms are concentrated. Most of the animals present in water mains are filter feeders or detritivores, and it could be expected that the microorganisms form a substantial proportion of the material ingested by the animals. Although a microbial flora may be present in the gut of the animals, it is likely that the predominant effect of the animals will be to exert a "grazing pressure" by ingesting and inactivating microorganisms. This may reduce the biomass of microbial material present, and may have a selective effect on the relative abundance of microbial species present. However, no studies have quantified either of these effects.

It has been noted that when control measures are applied against some species of animal in water distribution systems, the composition of the pipe fauna changes and other species increase. It is not known what effect such changes have on the composition of the biofilms.

6.3.4 Association between animals and pathogens

In natural waters, bacteria are present in the gut of various invertebrates and on their surfaces. This has led to speculation that, if the same were true of invertebrates in water supplies, this may be of sanitary significance. The microorganisms present in the guts of the invertebrates are likely to reflect those in the sediments and biofilms where they are feeding. In distribution systems carrying treated water, these would not normally be expected to include significant numbers of pathogens, and there is no reason to suppose that pathogens would be selectively favoured.

Viruses and parasites require specific hosts, and pathogenic bacteria generally require higher temperatures for multiplication than those found in water mains, at least in temperate countries. In the tropics, the situation may be different. Temperatures may be high enough to allow the proliferation of organisms such as Legionella, which multiplies above about 20°C. Legionella, which is infective through inhalation, has been isolated from protozoa (Lee & West, 1991); the possibility that it may also survive in macroinvertebrates cannot be discounted.

Among the few studies of the microflora associated with animals from water supplies, Levy, Hart and Cheetham (1986) took amphipods, insect larvae and copepods from samples from a distribution system in the USA. These animals were homogenised and the microflora studied. No enteric pathogens or coliforms were isolated in spite of the presence of coliforms in a service reservoir in the system. Some species which may be regarded as "opportunist" pathogens were identified: *Aeromonas*, *Pseudomonas*, *Serratia* and *Staphylococcus*. However, there is no evidence of any association of these organisms with waterborne gastrointestinal infection for the population at large (WHO 2003). Lupi, Ricci and Burrini (1995) examined the microflora of the guts of nematodes taken from a treated water supply and from the raw water from which it was derived. They found Enterobacteriaceae in the nematodes from both situations, although these bacteria were of nonpathogenic genera. Far fewer bacteria were found in the nematodes from the treated water.

6.3.5 Protection from disinfection

A few studies have suggested that invertebrates could harbour microorganisms in their gut and protect them from disinfection. Chang et al. (1960) conducted laboratory experiments using two species of nematode isolated from potable water in the USA and exposed to suspensions of microorganisms. They demonstrated that the nematodes would ingest *Salmonella* and *Shigella* bacteria, and coxsackie and echo viruses. A small proportion (around 1%) of these microorganisms survived in the gut of the nematodes for 48 hours. The nematodes were shown to be highly resistant to chlorination, and viable microorganisms were isolated from the gut after the nematodes were subject to chlorination. Chang et al. (1960) did not demonstrate the excretion of viable pathogens, but Smerda, Jensen and Anderson (1971) showed that viable *Salmonella* might be excreted by a nematode.

Levy et al. (1984) exposed amphipods to suspensions of *Escherichia coli* and *Enterobacter cloacae*, subjected them to chlorination (1 mg/l for 60 minutes), homogenized the animals and determined the count of viable bacteria. Viability of the bacteria in or on the amphipods was reduced to about 2% (*E. coli*) and 15% (*Enterobacter cloacae*). In contrast, bacteria that had not been in the presence of the amphipods were reduced to about 1% in 1 minute at this concentration of chlorine.

These studies demonstrated the possibility that invertebrates may protect microorganisms from disinfection, although they did not quantify the risks involved. It has not been demonstrated that pathogens have actually been present in a distribution system as a result of such a mechanism.

Theoretically, this mechanism could occur in the distribution system, although it would present a significant risk only if pathogens were already present in the distribution system and were protected from the levels of disinfectant carried through distribution. The microorganisms most likely to be protected in this way are those present in biofilms and sediments, which themselves offer protection from disinfection. It could be argued that grazing animals allow more effective penetration of disinfectant, by reducing the amount of organic matter present in biofilms and sediments. However, this theoretical possibility should not detract from the general objective of minimizing the formation of deposits and biofilms in the distribution system by appropriate treatment (Chapter 2) and routine maintenance (Chapter 4).

Another possibility raised by these studies is that some invertebrates could harbour microorganisms in water-treatment works, protect them from disinfection and carry them through treatment into the distribution system. This hazard only applies to the small numbers of animals passing treatment and not to the populations breeding in the distribution system. It represents a possible mechanism by which pathogens may be transported from a situation in which they may be relatively abundant (i.e. polluted raw water) to one in which otherwise they would be absent or rare (i.e. the treated water). Thus, the animals that warrant closer attention are likely to be those that appear to pass treatment more readily, such as chironomid larvae and nematodes. Again this risk is purely hypothetical and has not been observed in a piped-water supply system.

6.4 REMEDIAL MEASURES

6.4.1 Range of methods

The methods available for controlling existing infestations of animals in water mains include physical methods (essentially the mains cleaning techniques referred to in Chapter 4) and some chemical methods. The physical methods have the advantage of removing the sediments that provide habitat and food supply for animals, as well as the animals themselves. Effective application of the chemical methods also involves flushing. The most important of the chemical agents are pyrethroids, which are effective against a range of arthropods, including chironomid larvae and *Asellus*. Any chemical agent should be specifically approved for use in drinking-water (see WHO, 2004) Long-term control measures are recommended to restrict the potential for the growth of animal populations.

Regular monitoring of populations of animals in the distribution system, using the methods outlined in Section 6.2.2, will provide information on their relative abundance in different parts of the system and on changes in their numbers. This allows control measures to be taken pre-emptively in a planned manner at a time chosen by the water supplier, before numbers become high enough to cause major problems.

The choice of method adopted to control a particular infestation will depend on the species of animal present, whether consumers will tolerate them, their ease of removal and the numbers present. In general, species that move freely in the water or on the surface of the pipe or deposits (e.g. *Cyclops*) are relatively easily removed by flushing; whereas, those that burrow in deposits (e.g. nematodes, chironomid larvae) require action that is more stringent. Species that cling to the pipe surface (e.g. *Asellus*, aquatic gastropod snails) require dislodging before they can be flushed from the main.

Most of the methods involve the use of flowing water; they should be applied working systematically 'downstream', starting at the treatment works if practicable. No main that has been treated or is being treated should receive water from an untreated main. This is important to reduce recolonisation of cleaned mains; it requires accurate mains records and invariably involves several valving operations. For the methods to be effective, and to avoid unwanted side-effects, it is important that work is planned carefully and carried out thoroughly (see Section 4.4).

6.4.2 Physical methods

Systematic unidirectional flushing

Systematic flushing (see Section 4.4.2) removes most freely swimming animals, provided that adequate flows are available. In smooth pipes, it will also remove loose deposits and animals burrowing within them, but higher flows are required to achieve good results. Although most animals are of relatively low density, the pipe deposits often have a specific gravity of up to three; flows suitable for their removal should be used wherever possible. The solid particles transported by the water move more slowly than the water itself, so at least twice the nominal volume of water in the section of main should be flushed.

Swabbing

Swabbing (see Section 4.4.3) may be used where only moderate flows are available; it is generally effective at removing loose deposits and burrowing animals, and can also remove lightly attached organisms such as aquatic gastropod snails. However, swabbing is not very effective in badly encrusted mains.

Air scouring

Air scouring (see Section 4.4.4) may be used where only moderate pressures are available; it will effectively remove virtually all loose deposits and attached animals. It is less affected by encrustation on the pipe walls than foam swabbing. However, air scouring is normally restricted to mains up to 200 mm in diameter, and it may exacerbate corrosion in corroding iron mains.

6.4.3 Chemical methods

Chlorine

The concentrations of chlorine or chloramines normally found in water leaving treatment works, and that would be acceptable to consumers, are not very effective against most of the animals found in distribution systems. There is evidence that the higher concentrations that may be applied during water treatment have some effect in reducing animal penetration through treatment (Evins & Greaves, 1979). The oligochaete worms (e.g. *Nais*) are susceptible to moderate concentrations of chlorine; free chlorine concentrations raised to 0.5–1 mg/l, carried through the distribution system, have been used for control (Sands, 1969). Occasionally, very high concentrations of chlorine or chloramines have been used to counter particular problems after disconnecting consumers. For example, 12 mg/l chlorine has been used to kill leeches in a small isolated section of distribution system (Smalls & Greaves, 1968) and about 70 mg/l of chloramines has been used to kill chironomid larvae in temporarily isolated tanks (Broza et al., 1998).

Pyrethroids

Natural pyrethrins and a synthetic analogue, permethrin, have been used very successfully to control *Asellus*, other crustaceans such as *Gammarus*, and chironomid larvae (Burfield & Williams, 1975; Abram, Evans & Hobson, 1980; Mitcham & Shelley, 1980; Crowther and Smith, 1982). Although permethrin is chemically distinct from pyrethrins, it shares a number of properties that are important in its use for controlling animals in water mains. Among these are a very wide margin between the concentration that is effective in killing a range of aquatic animals, and the concentration that is toxic when drunk by mammals. For both substances the dose commonly used is 10 µg/l, which has not been considered a risk to consumers (Abram, Evans & Hobson, 1980; Fawell, 1987). The WHO guideline value for permethrin in drinking-water is 20 µg/l in the third edition of the WHO *Guidelines for Drinking-water Quality* (WHO, 2004). Because this value does not represent a significant risk to consumers over protracted periods of exposure, there is a significant margin of safety in comparison to the short periods for which permethrin may be present in drinking-water due to its occasional addition for control of animals. However, it is important that the dosing exercise is carefully controlled and monitored.

As the concentration effective for controlling animals in water mains is highly toxic to fish, it should not be discharged to watercourses, and warnings should be issued to those who may be affected (e.g. aquaculture, fisheries, aquaria). In some countries, the addition of pesticides to drinking-water is now prohibited and this precludes the use of pyrethrins or permethrin. In countries where the use of these chemicals is permitted, a decision to use them should take into account the seriousness of the infestation to be controlled and the available capacity to plan, control and monitor the operation. A carefully controlled and monitored application of these pesticides makes intensive use of technically qualified staff, and causes appreciable disruption to the system. Thus, it is only likely to be worthwhile to combat serious infestations. Note that these compounds are not included on the list of pesticides recommended by the WHO Pesticide Evaluation Scheme (WHOPES) for application to drinking-water sources for control of mosquito larvae for public health purposes (i.e. to control the disease vector).[1]

The preferred method of application is to treat an area that is small enough to allow systematic unidirectional flushing to be carried out in about 24 hours. The area should be separated from adjacent areas by closed valves to prevent reinfestation from untreated areas. Metered districts generally provide a convenient area, with adjacent areas treated subsequently. Consumers are not

---

[1] WHOPES documents can be obtained on request from the WHO Pesticide Evaluation Scheme, Communicable Disease Control, Prevention and Eradication, World Health Organization, 1211 Geneva 27, Switzerland.

usually disconnected. The pesticide solution is injected into a main under pressure at a rate proportional to the water flow. This ensures that, initially, all water flowing into the area being treated is at the target concentration, typically 10 µg/l. The network served from the point of injection is subject to systematic unidirectional flushing to draw the pesticide through the whole system. Twice the calculated volume in each length of main should be flushed. The pesticide tends to leave solution very readily (because of adsorption onto pipe surfaces and deposits); thus, some loss is to be expected as the water flows through the distribution system. It is advisable to monitor the concentrations reaching various points in the network during the dosing exercise. After allowing 24 hours contact, the dosing is discontinued and the systematic unidirectional flushing exercise is repeated to remove dead or moribund animals, and to draw fresh water into the system.

Other substances

In the past, some workers have suggested the use of copper for the control of animals in water mains, including *Asellus* and *Nais*, but its use has not found favour because it may promote corrosion of iron mains.

6.4.4 Measures suitable for different groups of animals

Isopoda

Isopoda are commonly known as 'slaters'. One example is *Asellus aquaticus*, which may be up to 15 mm long, so is obvious to consumers. It adapts readily to conditions in water mains and clings tenaciously to pipe walls. In a survey by van Lieverloo (1997) in the Netherlands, it comprised about 80% of the biomass of animals flushed from hydrants. Most complaints are received when the adult organisms die following reproduction in spring; at other times, large numbers may be present in the pipes without causing complaints. Collingwood (1964) suggested that the best season for control is in spring, immediately before the peak in reproduction. *Asellus* is controlled most effectively by dosing with pyrethrins or permethrin, accompanied by unidirectional systematic flushing of twice the pipe volume (see Section 6.4.3). Smaller crustaceans such as *Cyclops* and chydorids often increase after removal of *Asellus* using pyrethroids (Smalls, 1965). Both foam swabbing and air scouring may achieve moderately good removal of *Asellus* in favourable circumstances: they may also remove more sediments and thus inhibit reinfestation by other species.

Amphipoda

Amphipoda are freshwater shrimps; for example, *Gammarus*. *Gammarus* are up to about 15 mm long, so are obvious to consumers. Although they may be widespread, they seem not to increase to the densities shown by *Asellus*. They swim and are more easily removed by physical methods such as flushing and swabbing than *Asellus*. They are also susceptible to pyrethroids.

Insecta

Insecta are wormlike organisms; for example, the larvae of chironomids. Some species may be up to 25 mm long and bright red so are obvious to consumers, but most are much less conspicuous. Most species are unable to complete their life-cycle in the distribution system. They are controlled by systematic flushing or swabbing, depending on the flows available. Attention should be given to penetration of larvae through treatment works, access of adults to treatment works and ingress of adults through openings in service reservoirs. For those species that can complete their life-cycle in the distribution system, infestations can be successfully controlled using pyrethrins (Burfield & Williams, 1975) and permethrin (Mitcham and Shelley, 1980), where the use of these chemicals is permitted.

Oligochaeta (true worms) e.g. Nais

Worm species common in water mains are small and slender (typically up to 7 mm long and 0.3 mm wide), but may be noticed when they swim. Other aquatic species may be somewhat larger. They can be controlled by unidirectional systematic flushing, swabbing or air scouring, with the free chlorine concentration raised to 0.5 mg/l throughout the distribution system for a few weeks. The maintenance of a residual of 0.2 mg/l or more is likely to prevent reinfestation.

Nematoda

Nematoda, commonly known as roundworms, are plant parasites, animal parasites or free-living organisms that feed on organic matter. Most, but not all, are invisible to the naked eye. Those found in water mains are not easy to identify but are thought to be mainly small free-living aquatic species, thriving in locations that are rich in organic detritus. They can be controlled by flushing, swabbing or air scouring.

Gastropoda (aquatic snails)

Many of the gastropoda (aquatic snails) that are prevalent in water pipes are small (e.g. 5 mm long), although some are appreciably larger. They cling to pipe walls, so are not effectively removed by flushing. Foam swabbing is effective in pipes that are not badly encrusted. Although specific molluscicides are available for agricultural use, none are known to be suitable for use in potable water supplies.

Smaller crustacea

Smaller crustacea include species such as *Cyclops* and *Chydorus*. The *Cyclops* that are common in water mains are mostly about 1.5–2 mm long, although some are larger. They may be noticed by consumers because they dart jerkily through the water. The chydorids are less than 1 mm long, and are not noticed individually by consumers. However, they may occur in very large numbers, and cast their carapaces frequently. These may become iron stained and be seen by consumers as discoloured water. In general, these crustacea can be controlled by systematic flushing if flows are adequate, or by swabbing or air scouring.

6.4.5 Long-term control measures

Long-term control measures are recommended to prevent animals reaching nuisance levels or, following disinfestation, to prevent recurrence of problems. The principal objective is to deny the animals a food supply and to restrict their entry into the distribution system.

Removal of particulate organic matter at treatment works

Probably the single most important step in limiting animal populations in mains is to minimize the quantity of particulate organic matter entering the distribution system. Many algae are suitable as food for filter feeding animals, and they comprise the bulk of particulate organic matter in water derived from impounded surface sources. Different treatment processes are best suited to removing different types of algae: the processes should be selected and optimized to take account of the types of algae present.

Removal of assimilable organic matter at treatment works

Assimilable organic material may contribute to the growth of microorganisms, and thus indirectly to the growth of animals. Processes should be selected and operated to minimize the quantity of assimilable organic matter leaving the works, as discussed in Section 2.3.3.

Removal of animals at treatment works

Virtually all works treating surface waters allow the passage of some animals, although the numbers may be very small when compared with those in the raw water, and do not account for the numbers found in distribution. In general, coagulation and sedimentation are not effective at removing animals. Slow sand filtration appears to give better removal than rapid gravity filtration. Planktonic species, which predominate in stored waters, are relatively easily removed by treatment and do not thrive in the distribution system. Benthic species, which account for a greater proportion of the raw water community in river waters, are more likely to pass treatment, and in turn are more likely to thrive in the distribution system. Organisms that are able to burrow in particulate media, such as chironomid larvae, nematodes and oligochaete worms, seem well adapted to penetrate treatment, and significant numbers of chironomids have been found at all stages of treatment.

It is unusual for animal removal to be made a specific objective in the management of treatment works. Nevertheless, attention to such things as the effectiveness of backwashing is likely to be beneficial in this respect. In rapid sand filters, particular care should be taken to eliminate "dead spots" where the sand bed is not effectively fluidised. Prechlorination has been shown to help the removal of animals: this benefit should be balanced against other considerations, such as formation of disinfection by-products.

Measures taken in the distribution system

Certain "good housekeeping" practices carried out in the distribution system will limit the potential for animal infestations. Service reservoirs should be covered. Ventilators on these reservoirs should be covered with 0.5 mm mesh to exclude flying insects, overflows should be fitted with nonreturn valves and inspection covers should be tightly fitting. Unused dead end mains should be eliminated where practicable, and the size of mains should be appropriate for the flows to be carried because slow-flowing water is conducive to precipitation of solids and to animal growth. Hygienic precautions should be taken when repairing mains. Water pressure should be maintained to discourage ingress and contamination. Mains and service reservoirs should be routinely cleaned to remove particulate matter.

6.5 SUMMARY

Any supply of water containing visible living animals or animal debris will discourage consumption and encourage the use of alternative supplies that may have a better appearance but may be less safe. Thus, for reasons of public health, it is important to prevent the entry and proliferation of animals in water distribution networks.

Regular monitoring of the populations of animals in distribution systems allows control measures to be applied pre-emptively. A number of measures are available for limiting the populations of animals in water distribution systems. Short-term measures are mostly based on methods for cleaning solid material from the pipes. Some chemical methods are also available; however, there are restrictions on the use of these in some countries. Their use should be carefully controlled and monitored, and this requires intensive use of technically qualified staff. Long-term measures are mostly based on limiting the quantity of organic matter entering the distribution system and prevention of entry.

A small number of studies have demonstrated the possibility that invertebrates may protect microorganisms from disinfection. Within a distribution system carrying well-treated water, the risk of a significant number of pathogens being protected in this way is thought to be extremely small. The risk posed by invertebrates protecting microorganisms from disinfection during their passage through water treatment works is also likely to be very small. This mechanism is relatively unstudied and little understood.

6.6 REFERENCES

Abram FSH, Evins C, Hobson JA (1980). *Permethrin for the control of animals in water mains*. Technical Report TR 145, Water Research Centre, Medmenham, UK.

Berg MB (1995). Infestation of enclosed water supplies by chironomids (*Diptera: Chironomidae*): two case studies. In Cranston PS, ed. *Chironomids: from genes to ecosystems*. CSIRO Australia, East Melbourne, 241–246.

Broza M et al. (1998). Shock chloramination: potential treatment for *Chironomidae* (Diptera) larvae nuisance abatement in water supply systems. *Journal of Economic Entomology*, 91:834–840.

Burfield I, Williams DN (1975). Control of parthenogenetic chironomids with pyrethrins. *Water Treatment and Examination*, 24:57–67.

Chang SL et al. (1960). Survival, and protection against chlorination, of human enteric pathogens in free-living nematodes isolated from water supplies. *American Journal of Tropical Medicine and Hygiene*, 9(2):136–142.

Collingwood RC (1964). *Animals in distribution systems*. Technical Memorandum TM 27, Water Research Association, Medmenham, UK.

Crowther RF, Smith PB (1982). Mains infestations control using permethrin. *Journal of the Institution of Water Engineers and Scientists*, 36(3):205–214.

Evins C, Greaves GF (1979). *Penetration of water treatment works by animals*. Technical report TR 115, Water Research Centre, Medmenham, UK.

Evins C, Liebeschuetz J, Williams SM (1990). *Aesthetic water quality problems in distribution systems. A source document for the water mains rehabilitation manual*. Water Research Centre, Swindon, UK, 69–76, 139–151.

Fawell JK (1987). *An assessment of the safety in use of permethrin for disinfestation of water mains*. Report PRU 1412-M/1, Water Research Centre, Medmenham, UK.

Krüger F (1941). Parthenogenetische Stylotanytarsuslarven als Bewohner einer Trinkwasserleitung. *Archiv für Hydrobiologie*, 38(2):214–253.

Lee JV, West AA (1991). Survival and growth of *Legionella* species in the environment. Symposium supplement, *Journal of Applied Bacteriology*, 70:121S-129S.

Levy RV et al. (1984). Novel method for studying the public health significance of macroinvertebrates occurring in potable water. *Applied and Environmental Biology*, 47:889–894.

Levy RV, Hart FL, Cheetham RD (1986). Occurrence and public health significance of invertebrates in drinking water systems. *Journal of the American Water Works Association*, 78(9):105–110.

Lupi E, Ricci V, Burrini D (1995). Recovery of bacteria in nematodes from a drinking water supply. *Journal of Water Supply: Research and Technology — Aqua*, 44, pp 212–218.

Mitcham RP, Shelley MW (1980). The control of animals in water mains using permethrin, a synthetic pyrethroid. *Journal of the Institution of Water Engineers and Scientists,* 34:474–483.

Sands JR (1969). *The control of animals in water mains.* Technical Paper TP 63, Water Research Association, Medmenham, UK.

Smalls IC (1965). *Animals in a public water supply.* Technical Paper TP 49, Water Research Association, Medmenham, UK.

Smalls IC, Greaves GF (1968). A survey of animals in distribution systems. *Water Treatment and Examination,* 17:150–186.

Smart AC (1989). An investigation of the ecology of water distribution systems. PhD thesis, University of Leicester, UK.

Smerda SM, Jensen HJ, Anderson AW (1971). Escape of Salmonellae from chlorination during ingestion by *Pristonchus ihertheri* (*Nematoda Diplogasterinae*). *Journal of Nematology,* 3:201–204.

van Lieverloo H (1997). How to control invertebrates in distribution systems: by starvation or by flushing? *Proceedings of the American Water Works Association, Water Quality Technology Conference.* AWWA, Denver, USA.

WHO (1996). *Guidelines for drinking-water quality,* 2nd ed., vol. 2, *Health criteria and other supporting information.* Geneva, World Health Organization, 68–74.

Williams DN (1974). An infestation by a parthenogenetic chironomid. *Water Treatment and Examination,* 23(2):215–231.

WHO (2003). *Heterotrophic plate count measurement and drinking-water safety: the significance of HPCs for water quality and human health.* Eds Bartram J, Cotruvo J, Exner M, Fricker C, Glasmacher A. World Health Organization, Geneva, IWA Publishing.]

WHO (2004) *Guidelines for drinking-water quality,* 3rd ed. World Health Organization, Geneva.

7
Risk management for distribution systems

Melita Stevens, Guy Howard, Annette Davison, Jamie Bartram and Daniel Deere

7.1 INTRODUCTION

The safety of drinking-water depends on a number of factors, including quality of source water, effectiveness of treatment and integrity of the distribution system that transports the water to consumers. At every stage in the production and delivery of drinking-water, hazards can potentially compromise the quality of the water. Piped distribution systems may be less vulnerable to contamination than open surface-water catchments; however, if piped systems become contaminated, there may be no treatment processes to reduce risks from the introduced hazards.

The previous chapters have reviewed knowledge about the presence, growth and significance of microorganisms in piped networks. They have also

© 2004 World Health Organization. *Safe Piped Water: Managing Microbial Water Quality in Piped Distribution Systems.* Edited by Richard Ainsworth. ISBN: 1 84339 039 6. Published by IWA Publishing, London, UK.

described the operating practices of water supply organizations that can directly or indirectly influence the presence of microorganisms, especially those of significance to public health. However, this information is of little benefit unless it is part of a package of working practices designed to manage hazards in the whole supply system. Identifying, prioritizing and preventing risk arising from such hazards is the basis of a water safety plan approach. Such an approach is described in Chapter 4 of the latest edition of the World Health Organization's (WHO) *Guidelines for Drinking-Water Quality* (WHO, 2004). The remainder of this chapter demonstrates how control measures for distribution system can fit within a water safety plan.

7.2 WATER SAFETY PLANS

7.2.1 Elements of a water safety plan

Figure 7.1 describes development of a water safety plan. The objective of the plan is to supply water of a quality that will allow health-based targets to be met. The success of the plan is assessed through surveillance. The three central components of a water safety plan are:
- system assessment, which involves assessing the capability of the drinking-water supply chain (up to the point of consumption) to deliver water of a quality that meets the identified targets, and assessing design criteria for new systems
- identification of control measures in a drinking-water system that will collectively control identified risks and ensure that health-based targets are met (for each control measure identified, an appropriate means of monitoring should be defined that will ensure that any deviation from required performance is rapidly detected in a timely manner)
- management plans that describe actions to be taken during normal operation or extreme and incident conditions, and that document system assessment (including upgrade and improvement), monitoring, communication plans and supporting programmes.

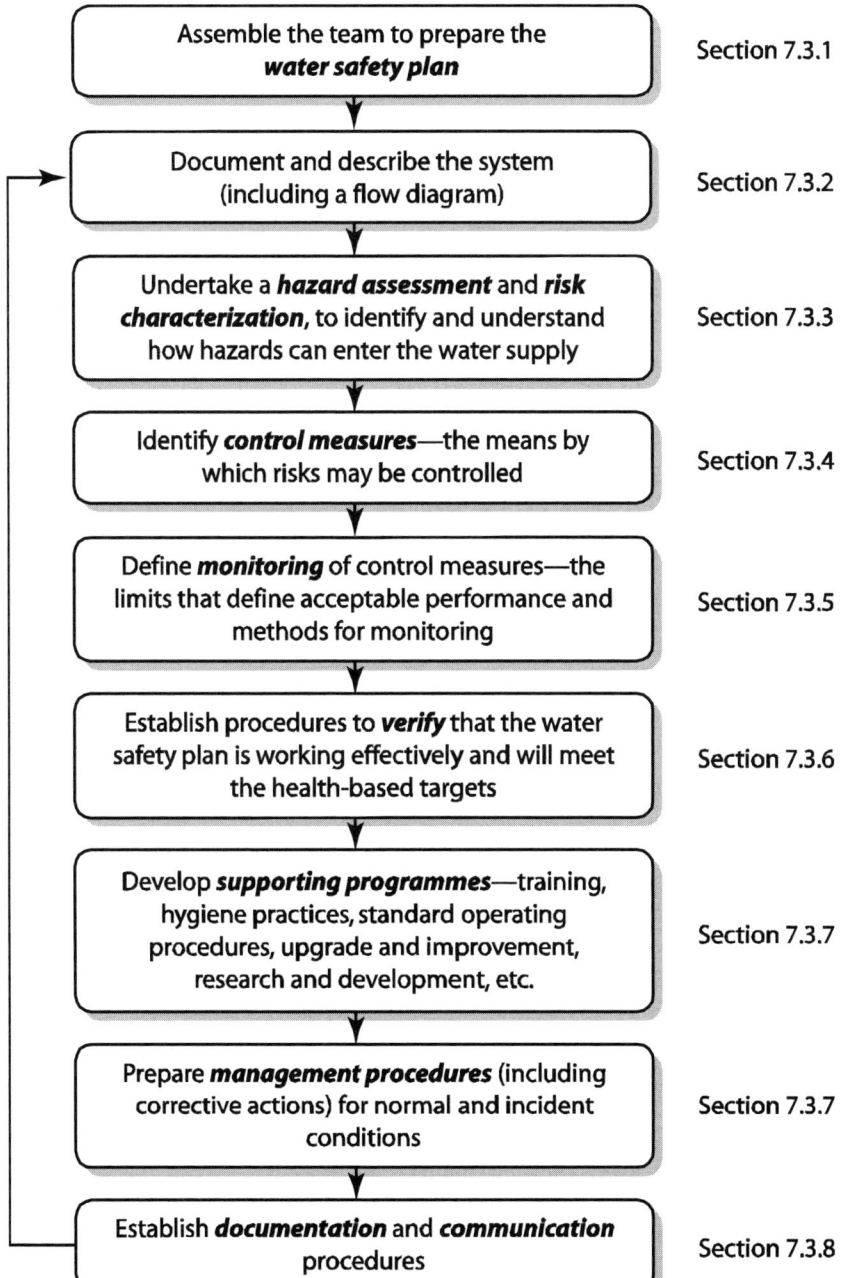

Figure 7.1. Overview of the water safety plan framework.

7.3 WATER SAFETY PLANS FOR DISTRIBUTION SYSTEMS

In general, water entering a drinking-water distribution system should be safe to drink, without additional treatment, once it has reached the first consumer connection. Therefore, the management of distribution systems primarily involves maintaining water quality, and minimizing the risk of contamination and deterioration of quality during transport. However, many distribution systems are a complex array of pipes, pumps, tanks and valves, which means that risks are not always as easily identified as in other areas of drinking-water supply.

7.3.1 Assemble team

The first step in developing a water safety plan is to assemble a multidisciplinary team with an understanding of the specific distribution system, to describe that system. The team would typically include managers, engineers (operations, maintenance, design and capital investment), water quality control staff (microbiologists and chemists) and technical staff involved in day-to-day operations. All members of the team should have a good knowledge of the system.

7.3.2 Document and describe the system

The next step is to document and describe the system. The description can include a basic flow diagram of the drinking-water distribution system, and reference to maps showing water quality networks and zones. It is important to capture the elements of the water supply system in sufficient detail to allow risks to be assessed and control measures to be identified. Therefore, pressure, pumps, connections, valves (and their status) and tanks need to be considered. Exmples of important features include:

- service reservoirs, balancing tanks, booster stations and (when used) break-pressure tanks
- zones of supply from each source
- layout of primary, secondary and tertiary pipelines (coded by colour or numerically)
- location of major valve boxes and junctions
- flow within the system (clearly indicated, noting where there are areas of interconnection between different zones)
- numbers of consumer connections
- hydraulic system flow rates and paths (including two-way flow)
- connections with high backflow hazard.

The representation of the system must be conceptually accurate, because the team will use the diagram as the basis for hazard analysis. If the flow diagram and system maps are incorrect, the team may miss potentially significant hazards, and may fail to identify existing or required control measures. Therefore, the team should validate the completeness and accuracy of the flow diagram and maps; for example, by visually checking against features observed on the ground. Proof of validation is typically recorded, together with an accountability (e.g. a member of the team may sign and date a flowchart and a set of maps to validate that they are accurate and complete).

The example given in Box 7.1 (below) illustrates the importance of being aware of the major components of the distribution system.

7.3.3 Hazard assessment and risk characterization

Managing risks in distribution systems poses different challenges to managing risks in, for example, a treatment plant. When considering engineered treatment processes such as filtration and disinfection, the emphasis is on selecting and controlling processes that will reduce risk to an acceptable level, assuming that the source water has potentially unacceptable contamination. When considering distribution systems, the focus is on preventing recontamination or degradation of water quality caused by breaches in system integrity or difficult operational circumstances. In both situations, it is useful to determine what contaminants are of concern (hazard assessment), and how they may reach unacceptable levels (risk characterization). This makes it easier to identify important potential contaminants (hazards) and the risk of events occurring that could cause these hazards to contaminate the system (hazardous events).

Risk management in distribution systems is similar to that in catchments, in that the aim is to prevent the introduction of hazards. However, a major difference is that distribution systems represent the final barrier before consumption in many supplies, whereas hazards arising in catchments may be reduced during storage and treatment.

In risk assessment, it is important to be explicit about the risks that are to be assessed, in terms of who is at risk, and what they are at risk from. Therefore, the following questions are helpful as a first step in risk assessment:
- How is the water to be used and what exposure routes are relevant?
- What consumer education is in place for water use?
- How are consumers notified of potential contamination?
- Who is the water intended for?
- What special considerations are in place for vulnerable groups such as infants, the elderly and the immunocompromised?

> **Box 7.1.** Outbreak of Norwalk virus caused by a cross connection between a municipal supply and a private supply.
>
> During one week in August 1980, approximately 1500 people from a small community in the north of the State of Georgia, USA, developed gastroenteritis. Stool culture was negative for *Salmonella*, *Shigella* and *Campylobacter*. Only four stool samples were examined by electron microscopy and these were negative. However, 12 of 19 paired sera showed a fourfold rise in titre of antibody to norovirus, confirming the diagnosis. A door-to-door survey of households revealed marked variation in reported attack rates, with the highest attack rate (68%) in people living close to a textile plant. Epidemiological investigation also found an association between illness and consumption of tap water.
>
> Within the affected area there were two water supplies — a nearby river and a spring source. There was no relevant illness in people whose water was supplied from the river source; those who were affected by the outbreak had received water sourced from the spring
>
> The spring source, which was chlorinated, was found be satisfactory and the chlorination plant to be working adequately. There were, however, two known connections between this municipal water system and a private system supplying water to a textile plant. The water for the textile plant came from five wells and two springs in the area. Each source was chlorinated, though the chlorination equipment was antiquated and inadequate. One of the springs was contaminated with high counts of total and thermotolerant coliforms, and storage reservoirs for the textile plant water were grossly contaminated with algae and pinnate diatoms.
>
> The water pressure in the municipal system (110 psi) was normally higher than in the textile plant system (100 psi). However, demands on the municipal system sometimes reduced the pressure to only 80 psi, which would have allowed substantial flow of water from the textile plant system to the municipal system.
>
> The outbreak illustrates the importance of avoiding cross connections between systems where the water utility does not have complete control of the water quality of both systems.
>
> Source: Kaplan et al. (1982).

Desktop risk assessment

The next step in risk assessment is to systematically evaluate the system's potential vulnerability to external hazards, using the flow diagrams and system maps. The initial evaluation is desk-based and relies on data supplied by design and operational staff.

Information that would normally be part of this assessment includes the following:
- areas where (possibly seasonal) soil moisture content or flooding makes it likely that faecal matter from sources on the surface or shallow subsurface will enter the system
- any other sources of faecal matter found in the urban area (e.g. animal husbandry)
- areas of high population density (used as a surrogate for faecal loading in the environment)
- areas of low pressure within the system
- areas of intermittent supply and their likely recharging pattern
- pipe material, age and condition (a vulnerability score can be developed based on likely risk of breaks or joint failure)
- cross-connections, proximity to sewers and high-hazard facilities, and the relative depth of water supply pipes and sewers
- low-lying areas prone to flooding
- depth to which pipes are buried (this differs from the point above concerning sewers, because it relates to the risk of accidental breakage by traffic, etc)
- condition and age of service reservoirs
- areas where there are significant numbers of illegal connections or where the tertiary infrastructure has been installed by nonutility staff and quality of construction is uncertain
- areas where a significant proportion of houses use household storage, which may include the attachment of small pumps to the main, for pumping to roof tanks
- areas of known high leakage
- large buildings, such as hospitals.

At each step, the objective is to identify how contamination could arise from the identified hazards, by considering the events that could lead to the presence of contamination. The output from this exercise is a list of hazardous events, their associated hazards and a reference to where in the system or process the risks are located.

Sanitary survey

The above steps provide an overall picture of the distribution system and a framework for identifying hazardous environments and vulnerability. The next step is to carry out a field assessment of the system, to identify potential hazards and hazardous events, and the existence of possible control measures (described in Section 7.3.4).

The sanitary survey gathers field evidence to support the risk assessment. It involves systematic investigation of the complete distribution system, to identify all major hazards and vulnerable points. The survey deals mainly with the physical state of infrastructure, focusing primarily on external threats.

In undertaking a sanitary survey, standard forms can be used for major structures of the same type, such as service reservoirs, major valve boxes, road or culvert crossings and distribution infrastructure. Standardized forms for sanitary surveys and inspections are available (WHO, 1997; Howard, 2002), and can help to ensure that the importance of different major components of the system is evaluated, and persistent failures identified.

Urban piped water supplies can be difficult to survey, because most sanitary inspections are based on observation. Leaks associated with deep-laid pipes are often difficult to detect through observation, and contamination may occur a significant distance from a sample site. However, simple visual and question-based approaches can still provide useful information about whether risks are at the level of the general supply or are localized. Thus, questions on the inspection form should deal both with risks found in the immediate area and those that relate to broader supply problems. Local risks will include aspects such as the pooling of stagnant water around the joints between riser pipes and delivery mains. Tap leakage, pipe exposure and waste allowed to collect around the tap may be significant causes of contamination. Inspections are required at service reservoirs because these have the potential to cause widespread contamination.

There are difficulties of scale in a comprehensive sanitary inspection of an entire urban piped water system. The areas to be inspected by field staff should be broken down into segments that can be easily covered within one day — this may be a full water supply zone or an acceptable subdivision.

The importance of having an understanding of the vulnerability of a distribution system is illustrated by the example given in Box 7.2 (below).

Prioritizing risks

In large and complex systems, so many risks may be identified that it is difficult to set priorities. Simple matrices for risk assessment typically combine technical information from guidelines, scientific literature and industry practice with well-informed "expert" judgement, supported by third-party peer review or benchmarking. The risk ranking will be specific for any particular water supply system because each system is unique.

> **Box 7.2** Cryptosporidiosis associated with contamination of a water conduit.
>
> During August and September 2000, there were 168 laboratory confirmed case of cryptosporidiosis in residents of Belfast. Of these cases, 117 lived within the area supplied by a single water conduit. This drinking-water conduit had been built 110 years earlier. It was seven miles long and supplied drinking-water to some 216 000 people. The water passing through the conduit came from a water treatment works and was not further treated before being supplied to a number of distribution reservoirs and then consumers.
>
> Initial sampling of the water was negative for *Cryptosporidium* oocysts, although several large-volume samples taken from the service reservoirs were positive, with counts of up to 2.2 oocysts per 10 litres. To further investigate the integrity of the conduit, chlorination was turned off at the water treatment works and samples for total coliforms and *E. coli* taken at various points of the conduit through pre-existing airwells. Counts of total coliforms and *E. coli* increased substantially between two sampling points. Close-circuit television (CCTV) cameras were put into the conduit between these points. CCTV demonstrated black staining of the roof of the conduit, which was subsequently shown to coincide with the location of a private septic tank. On further inspection it was found that the outer brick wall of the conduit had been removed to enable the outflow of the septic tank to be constructed. Consequently, the overflow from the septic tank could contaminate the drinking-water distribution system after the treatment stage.
> Source: Department of Public Health Medicine(2001).

By using a semiquantitative risk assessment, the water safety plan team can calculate a priority score for each hazardous event identified. The objective is to focus on the most significant hazards and hazardous events, to begin to identify what might be the most important control measures (Section 7.3.4). Several approaches to ranking risk are available, and the team needs to determine which approach it will use. An example of an approach is given in Table 7.1, where the risk score for a particular hazardous event is determined by combining the likelihood of its occurrence with the severity of the consequences.

Table 7.2 gives examples of descriptors that coulc be used to rate the likelihood and severity for calculation of the risk score; other descriptors might be more appropriate in some situations.

In developing a water safety plan, it is possible to adopt an approach of continuous improvement, taking more risks into consideration at each iteration of the plan. To do this, the team needs to determine a cut-off point to distinguish between hazards that require immediate attention and those that can be considered in future iterations.

Table 7.1. Example of a simple risk scoring table for prioritizing risks.

	Severity of consequences				
	Insignificant	Minor	Moderate	Major	Catastrophic
Likelihood					
Almost certain	5	10	15	20	25
Likely	4	8	12	16	20
Moderate	3	6	9	12	15
Unlikely	2	4	6	8	10
Rare	1	2	3	4	5

Source: Davison et al. (2002)

Table 7.2. Examples of definitions of likelihood and severity categories for risk scoring.

Item	Definition	Weighting
Likelihood		
Almost certain	Once a day	5
Likely	Once per week	4
Moderate	Once per month	3
Unlikely	Once per year	2
Rare	Once every 5 years	1
Severity		
Catastrophic	Potentially lethal to large population	5
Major	Potentially lethal to small population	4
Moderate	Potentially harmful to large population	3
Minor	Potentially harmful to small population	2
Insignificant	No impact or not detectable	1

7.3.4 Control measures

In the context of a water safety plan, a control measure is any action or activity that can be used to prevent or eliminate a hazard, or reduce it to an acceptable level. Therefore, any risk management activity in a drinking-water supply is considered to be a control measure. Examples of control measures in water distribution are positive pressure, intact pipe networks, backflow preventers and vermin proofing on tanks.

Control measures are identified by considering the events that can cause contamination of water, both directly and indirectly, and the activities that can mitigate the risks from those events. Examples of control measures in the distribution system include:

- maintenance of the distribution system

Risk management

- availability of backup systems (e.g. power supply)
- maintenance of an adequate disinfectant residual
- presence of devices to prevent cross-connection and backflow
- use of fully enclosed distribution system and storages
- maintenance of a disinfection residual
- appropriate repair procedures, including disinfection of water mains after repairs
- maintenance of adequate system pressure
- maintenance of security to prevent sabotage, illegal tapping and tampering.

In identifying control measures, operational criteria to differentiate acceptable from unacceptable performance are required. These criteria, referred to as "operational limits", are control measure variables that can be measured (either directly or indirectly) or factors that can be observed. Examples of measurable variables include minimum and maximum values for pH, chlorine residuals or hydraulic system pressure at strategic locations in the distribution system; an example of a factor that can be observed is the apparent integrity of vermin-proofing screens on reservoirs. Current knowledge and expertise (including industry standards and technical data), and locally derived historical data can be used as a guide when determining the limits. Ideally, operational limits have the following properties:

- they can be defined and monitored (either directly, or indirectly through surrogates)
- a predetermined response (i.e. a corrective action, described in Section 7.3.5) can be implemented when monitoring indicates that conditions have deviated from set limits
- the corrective action will protect water safety by either bringing the control measure back within acceptable limits or causing additional control measures to be implemented
- the process of detecting deviation from limits and of responding will be sufficiently rapid to maintain water safety.

Control measures that cannot be defined, but meet the other requirements listed above, can still be important and can form part of the water safety plan.

7.3.5 Monitoring to support risk management

There are three kinds of monitoring in the management of distribution systems — operational, process validation and verification — each of which has a different purpose, as shown in Table 7.3. This section considers operational monitoring; Section 7.3.6 looks at monitoring for process validation and verification.

Table 7.3. Types of monitoring in the management of distribution systems

Monitoring type	Purpose
Operational	Support management of the operation of the system, to ensure safety and to ensure that control measures are working effectively
Process validation	Demonstrate that control measures are capable of achieving the required outcomes
Verification	A final check that the entire water supply system is functioning correctly

Operational monitoring and selection of operational control parameters

Operational monitoring involves conducting a planned sequence of observations or measurements, designed to assess whether the control measures applied at a point in the system are achieving their objectives. Effective monitoring relies on establishing what will be monitored, how, when and by whom. In most cases, routine operational monitoring will be based on simple surrogate observations or tests, such as turbidity or structural integrity, rather than complex microbial or chemical tests (which are likely to form part of process validation and verification, Section 7.3.6).

An essential requirement of operational monitoring is the ability to assess performance of the system in a timely manner, and judge whether a control measure is functioning properly. Microbial parameters (e.g. indicator bacteria) are of limited use for this purpose, because the time taken to process and analyse water samples is too slow (although changes in heterotrophic plate counts can be used to monitor the effectiveness of control measures for limiting biofilm activity or maintaining system integrity). Generally, operational monitoring for control measures such as pressure and levels can be online and in real time, although this is not always essential.

If monitoring shows that an operational or critical limit has been exceeded, then there is the potential for water to be, or to become, unsafe. The objective is to monitor control measures according to a statistically valid sampling plan and in a timely manner, to prevent the supply of any potentially unsafe water. A permanent record of monitoring should be maintained. For example, if chlorine disinfection is being used as a control measure for a distribution system, the parameters monitored could be chlorine residuals, established for the given system at particular set points (generally in parts per million, ppm). A range of values would be included, again calculated for the system, outside of which an alarm would be set to sound via a telemetry system. Since pH and turbidity are integral to chlorine efficacy, these parameters might also be monitored. Should the telemetry system show that the disinfection control measure was not within acceptable bounds, a pager system could be used to alert water quality personnel. These staff would then take predetermined corrective actions to investigate the deviation and bring the water back into specification, as discussed in the next section.

Establish corrective action for deviations that may occur

A corrective action is the action to be taken when the results of monitoring at a control point indicate a loss of control. For example, the ability to change temporarily to alternative water sources is one of the most useful corrective actions, although this option is not always available. Corrective actions should be specific and predetermined where possible, so that they can be employed rapidly. To allow for unforeseen events for which there may be no predetermined corrective action, a general incident and emergency response plan should be developed, to at least set up a response framework. By ensuring that a contingency is available in the event of an operational limit being exceeded, safety of supply can be maintained.

The following are examples of possible corrective actions that could be taken when online monitoring of chlorine disinfection fails to comply with operational limits (all of these corrective actions would include action from the on-call or designated water quality personnel):

- ensure that the telemetry system is working and that the alarm is not false
- review or adjust the range of chlorine residuals, and increase the chlorine dosing level if necessary
- flush any undisinfected water from the main
- make any necessary repairs or operational control changes.

Communication is a crucial component of corrective actions. Therefore, a procedure for notifying sensitive customers (e.g. hospitals) and authorities (e.g. health departments) should be included in corrective actions. For example, it may be necessary to have an understanding with a local bottled water company, to ensure that residential customers at least receive drinking water in the event of a distribution system failure.

7.3.6 Verification

Verification is the final check of water safety. It provides an objective confirmation of the overall safety of the system. For example, biophysical verification activities, such as microbial and chemical monitoring, are likely to be undertaken in the distribution system. Verification also encompasses audit and review of the water safety plan, including checking compliance with operational procedures.

Verification monitoring involves using methods, procedures or tests, in addition to, and independent of, those used in operational monitoring, to determine whether the water safety plan:
- complies with the stated objectives outlined in the water quality targets
- needs modification and revalidation
- is controlling the identified hazard.

Verification monitoring may be less frequent than operational monitoring. For example, operational monitoring might be online (and thus continuous) through a telemetry system, whereas verification monitoring of distribution storage tanks and reservoirs might be carried out fortnightly.

Bacterial indicators, such as *E. coli*, are the indicator most frequently used for final verification of microbiological quality. Although microbial monitoring can be used in verification as a final check, end-point testing should not be relied on for operational control because, by the time samples have been processed and analysed, water will already have been treated and delivered to consumers.

Auditing of compliance with the water safety plan is another form of verification. The objective is to assess the extent to which the plan is being followed in practice. Auditing may involve both internal and external auditors, and may include review of important activities related to water safety, such as compliance with operational procedures, adoption of training plans and timely calibration of equipment. An example of a verification schedule is given in Table 7.4.

Table 7.4. Example of verification schedule for calibration of equipment.

Activity	Description	Frequency	Person responsible	Records
Calibration of equipment	Analysing and testing equipment to be maintained and calibrated according to maintenance schedules	According to maintenance schedules	Laboratory technician, operators	Laboratory calibration records

Process validation

Process validation involves obtaining evidence that the elements of the water safety plan will be effective. An example of such validation is the provision of objective evidence that a control measure, operating within its operational limits, will control the relevant hazard. Validation can be based on a variety of sources, including the scientific literature, trade associations, regulation and legislation, historical data, professional bodies and suppliers.

System-specific validation is essential, because variations in water or system design may have a large impact on the efficacy of certain control measures. Thus, a control measure that works in one distribution system may be less effective in another type of distribution system. Examples of process validation are:
- modelling of flow paths in storage tanks to validate the extent of mixing
- measurement of conditions for effective disinfection in storage tanks
- measurement of microbial parameters, such as heterotrophic bacteria and coliforms (in this situation, the lag time for return of results from culture-based methods can be tolerated, because this type of monitoring is not used to support the day-to-day management of water safety).

The water safety plan should be reviewed at predetermined periods to incorporate new information as it becomes available, and to ensure that the plan is still capable of controlling the identified hazards.

7.3.7 Supporting programmes and management procedures

The delivery of safe water through a water safety plan involves managing people and processes. Therefore, adequate supporting programmes, such as training, supplier quality assurance and good hygiene practices, are an important part of the plan. Supporting programmes are activities that are essential for effective operation of control measures and that indirectly support water safety. Actions required to operate the system according to the water safety plan need to be captured in the form of management procedures, such as standard operating procedures. Management procedures should be developed for both routine and incident and emergency conditions.

7.3.8 Documentation

Records are essential for reviewing the adequacy and implementation of the water safety plan. Four types of records can be kept:
- support documentation for development of the water safety plan
- records generated by the water safety plan system
- documentation of methods and procedures used
- records of employee training programmes.

Records demonstrating adherence to the water safety plan are needed to support the verification auditing activities. In the short term, tracking of records allows an operator or manager to become aware that a process is approaching its operational limits, and review of records can help to identify trends so that operational adjustments can be made. In the long term, periodical review of records allows trends to be noted, so that appropriate actions can be determined and implemented, to ensure continual improvement.

Documentation is an essential part of following the water safety plan; it is also a powerful way of demonstrating that all due diligence and reasonable precautions have been taken by the utility, because the information is readily available, readily trackable and transparent.

7.5 SUMMARY OF WATER SAFETY PLAN CONTENT

Table 7.5 summarises the suitable content of a water safety plan, with the elements categorised as "must contain", "should contain" or "may contain".

Table 7.5. Summary of requirements of a water safety plan.

Must contain:
- process flow diagrams and maps, including identifying control measures
- hazard identification
- water safety plan document
- identification of water safety plan team
- description of the water supply, intended use and vulnerability
- documented contingency plans.

Should contain:
- supplier agreement documents
- detailed specifications for chemicals and materials used in the water supply
- job descriptions for those holding principal accountabilities for operating the water distribution system
- corrective action plans for deviations
- record-keeping procedures
- validation data
- procedures for verification and revision
- documented incident procedure.

May contain:
- relevant manuals such as for line hygiene, preventative maintenance, and equipment calibration measurements
- job descriptions and accountabilities for all staff
- training programme and records for all staff
- findings and corrective actions from previous audits (including verification procedures)
- consumer complaint policy and procedure.

7.6 REFERENCES

Davison A et al. (2002). *Water safety plans. Protection of the human environment.* Water, Sanitation and Health, World Health Organization, Geneva (WHO/SDE/WSH/02.09).

Department of Public Health Medicine (2001). *Report of an outbreak of cryptosporidiosis during August and September 2000 in the Lisburn, Poleglass and Dunmurry areas of the Eastern Board.* Eastern Health and Social Services Board, Belfast.

Howard G (2002). *Urban water supply surveillance — a reference manual.* Water, Engineering and Development Centre/Department for International Development, Loughborough University, UK.

Kaplan JE et al. (1982). Gastroenteritis due to Norwalk virus: an outbreak associated with a municipal water system. *Journal of Infectious Diseases*, 146:190–197.

WHO (2004) *Guidelines for drinking-water quality*, 3rd ed. World Health Organization, Geneva.

Index

abrasive swabs 77
Acanthamoeba 7
Aeromonas 6–7
aesthetics
   animal infestations 102, 108, 118
   metazoan animals 108
   microorganisms 2
   source mixing effects 54–5
aggressive cleaning 76–7
air gaps 62, 64
air scouring
   animal infestations 113
   pipe network cleaning 76, 79, 81, 83–4
air vessels 44–5
amoebae 7
amphipoda 111, 115–16
animal infestations 7–8, 101–19

AOC *see* assimilable organic carbon
approval systems, pipe materials 58–9
aquatic animals 104, 106–7, 112, 115
aquatic snails 116
Arizona 61
Asellus aquaticus 106, 107, 112, 115
assemble teams 124
assimilable organic carbon (AOC) 27–8, 32, 117
auditing 133, 134

backflow
   design 41–2, 59, 60, 62–5, 67
   hazard ratings 63–4
   health checklists 67
   Norwalk virus 75
   operation 41–2, 59, 60, 62–5, 67
   piped network hydraulics 41–2

bacteria
　microbiology 7–9
　prevention/minimization 21–30
bacteriological sampling 97
baffles 48
ball-type hydrants 42
BDOC *see* biodegradable dissolved organic carbon
Belfast 129
benthic species 104–5
BFP *see* biofilm formation potential
bilharziasis 109
biodegradable dissolved organic carbon (BDOC) 27–8, 32
biofilm formation potential (BFP) 28–9
biofilms
　animal population sizes 107
　formation 6–7, 11, 28–9
　growth factors 20–1
　monochloramine residual disinfection 25
　pathogenic microorganisms 8–9
　source mixing effects 56
biological nitrification 30
biological sand filters 31
booster chlorination 33, 50–2, 94
break tanks 62, 64
breeding populations 105, 106
Bristol, England 98
broken water mains 88, 98
by-passes 43

calcium hypochlorite 94
calibrating equipment 134
Campylobacter species 8
Canada 32
catchment protection 5
CCTV *see* close-circuit television
check valves 63, 64
chemical cleaning 73
chemical remedial measures, animal infestations 113–15
chironomid (gnat) larvae 105, 112
　remedial measures 113, 116, 117
chloramines 22, 23–4, 113
chlorination 33, 50–2, 94
chlorine
　animal infestations 113
　concentration/contact times 95–6
　construction/repair works 94–6
　residuals 11, 33
　treated water microbial quality 22–3
chlorine dioxide 22, 24
cholera 4
Chyodorus 117
clarifiers 31
cleaning
　construction/repair works 91–6
　frequency 73
　pipe networks 76–84
　service reservoirs and tanks 71, 73
Clitheroe Lancashire, England 10
close-circuit television (CCTV) 129
closed valves 57
coagulant residuals 26
coliform counts 11–13, 15, 32
communication in operational monitoring 133
community-managed systems 97–8
conduits 129
configurations of service reservoirs 47–8
connections 70
　see also cross-connections
construction
　materials 66–7
　precautions 87–99
　repair works guidelines 87–99
consumer relations 79
control measures 122, 127, 130–1
control valves 42–3, 62–3, 64, 65
controlling microorganisms 11
copper 115
Coquitlam, Canada 32
corrective actions 133
corrosion 8, 29–30
coxsackie 110–11

Index

cross-connections
  design 59–62, 63–4, 67
  hazard ratings 62, 63–4
  health checklists 67
  Norwalk virus 75, 126
  operation 59–62, 63–4, 67
crustacea 117
cryptosporidiosis 129
Cryptosporidium oocysts 10
Cyclops 8, 108–9, 117
Cyclops albidus 106

DCDA *see* double check detector assemblies
dead-ends 39–40, 57
decentralized treatments 33
deposits 56, 77, 103–4
depth of water 47
design and operation
  backflow protection 41–2, 59, 60, 62–5, 67
  chlorination stations 50–3
  cross-connection protection 59–62, 63–4, 67
  disinfectant residuals 50–3
  distribution systems 38–67
  health checklists 65–7
  mixing conditions 53–6
  pipe location 59
  pipe materials 58–9
  piped networks 39–46
  service reservoirs 46–50
  zoning networks 57–8
desktop risk assessments 126–7
detritivores 106
dichloramine 23–4
dimensions of service reservoirs 47
disinfectant residuals
  booster dosing 50–2
  design/operation 50–3
  health checklists 66
  management 25
  microbial quality 22

microbiology 11
  source mixing effects 55–6
disinfection
  animal associations 110–11, 119
  concentration/contact time 22–6
  construction/repair works 91–6
  water quality deterioration 32
dissolved organic carbon (DOC) 27–8
distribution systems
  animals 101–19
  biofilm formation 6–7
  construction/repair works 87–99
  design 38–67
  maintenance procedures 69–85
  microbial monitoring 12–14
  microorganisms 1–15
  mixing conditions 53–6
  operation 38–67
  risk management 121–36
  survey procedures 69–85
diving cleaning equipment 73
DOC *see* dissolved organic carbon
documentation
  repair works 88
  water safety plans 124–5, 135–6
double acting air valves 42
double check detector assemblies (DCDA) 63
double check valves 63
double-acting air valves 44–5
Dracunculus medinensis 8, 108
drinking-water
  animals 101–19
  microbial quality 30–2
  pathogens 6
dual check valves 63, 64

echo viruses 110–11
emergency repairs 89, 95, 97
engineering works 87–99
England *see* United Kingdom
enteric viruses 9

Enterobacter cloacae 111
environmental impacts 78–9
equipment
  calibration 134
  chlorination stations 51–2
Escherichia coli 12–13, 15, 111
Escherichia coli O157:H7 4–5, 8
excessive capacity 39
external examinations 71–2
external hazard vulnerability 126–7

faecal pollution 12–13, 61
feedback 52
field disinfection 94–6
field testing 64–5
filter-papers, colour 77
filtration 10–11, 31
fittings 70–1, 74–5, 84
fixed biomass proliferation 28–9
flocculation 30–1
flow
  conditions 56
  isolation fittings 74–5
  patterns 48–9
  proportional dosing 52
  rates 80
  surges 44–5
flushing
  animal infestations 112–13, 114–15
  pipe network cleaning 76, 79, 80–1
flying insects 105, 112
food-chains 7–8, 106
foxes 90
free living amoebae 7
frequency of inspection and cleaning 73
freshwater shrimps 115–16

GAC *see* granular activated carbon
Gammarus 115–16
gaseous dosing 52
gastropoda 116
Georgia, USA 126

giardiasis 61, 98
gnats *see* chironomid larvae
granular activated carbon (GAC) filtration 31
grazer populations 106, 107
growth
  biofilms 6–7, 11, 20–1, 28–9
  microorganisms 6–8, 20–1
guidelines
  construction/repair works 87–99
  microbiological parameters 12–13
guinea worm 8, 108

hazard assessments 125–30
hazard ratings 62, 63–4
health checklists 65–7
Helicobacter pylori 8
hepatitis 41
heterotrophic plate counts (HPC) 13
households, microbiology 9–11
HPC *see* heterotrophic plate counts
hydrants 42, 43, 44–5, 74–5
hydraulics 25, 39–42
hygiene training 97–8
hygienic safety 87–99
hypochlorous acid 22–3

India 88
ingress of animals 104–6
inlets 48
insect larvae 105, 112
  remedial measures 113, 116, 117
insecta 116
insects 105
inserted liners 92
inspection frequency 73
installation location/depth 43, 59
integrated operations 45–6
intermittent supply 41–2
internal...
  corrosion 29–30
  examinations 71, 72, 73
  surface cleaning 73

invertebrates 101–19
isolation 57–8
isopoda 115

jaundice 88
joints 70

laboratory testing 54, 56
large buildings 9–11
larvae 105, 112
   remedial measures 113, 116, 117
Legionella 6, 7, 110
Legionnaires' disease 25
liners 92
liquid dosing 52
location/siting
   chlorination stations 51
   pipes 59, 66–7
loops 39–40
loss of supply 49
low-flow dead-ends 39–40

mains
   cleaning programs 76–84, 92
   repair guidelines 92–3
maintenance 69–85
   access to piped networks 43
   backflow prevention 64–5
   chlorination stations 52
   cleaning 71, 73, 76–84
   pipes 75–9
   service reservoirs 70–5, 84
management safety plan procedures 122, 135
Massachusetts, USA 41
mechanical control valves 62–3, 64
mechanical scraping 76
membrane retention 32
metazoan animals 7–8, 108–12
metered services 65
microbial
   flora 109

growth factors 20–1
monitoring 12–14
quality
   animal effects 109
   source mixing effects 55–6
   treated water 19–34
safety 2–3
microflora 110
microorganisms 1–15
   animal associations 109–11
   construction/repair works 87–8
   control 11
   disinfection protection 110–11, 119
   growth 6–8, 20–1
   pathogens 8–9, 87, 88
   treatment plants 5–6
minimizing bacterial proliferation 21–30
Missouri, USA 4–5
mixing conditions 46–7, 53–6
modelling
   disinfectant residuals 25
   mixing conditions 53–4
   piped network hydraulics 40
   zoning networks 58
monitoring
   animal populations 118
   construction/repair works 96–7
   microbial safety 2–3
   pipe network cleaning 79
   risk management support 131–5
monochloramine 23–4, 25
Mycobacterium avium complex 6, 7

Naegleria 7
Naegleria Fowleri 7
Nais 113, 115, 116
negative pressures 40, 70
nematoda
   disinfection protection 110–11, 119
   parasitic 8, 108
   remedial measures 116

Netherlands 102
new supply introduction
　cleaning/disinfection 92
　mixing effects 54–5
nitrification 30
nitrogen trichloride 23–4
non-aggressive cleaning 76, 77–8, 79–84
nonreturn valves 42–3
Norwalk virus 75, 126
nutrients 21

oligochaete worms 113, 115, 116
operation and design *see* design and operation
operational limits 131
operational monitoring 131–3, 134
organic matter 27–9, 106–7
outlets 48
oxygen 21
ozone 22

parasites, viruses 110
parasitic flat worms 109
parasitic nematodes 8, 108
Paratanytarsus grimmii 105
particulate content 26
particulate organic matter 107, 117
pathogens
　animal associations 110
　microbiology 6–7, 8–9
　microorganism contamination 8–9, 87, 88
personnel 90–1
Peru, South America 4
pesticides 114–15
pH factors 21
physical remedial measures 112–13
Pierce County, Washington State, USA 75
pipe location 59, 66–7
pipe materials 9, 58–9, 66–7, 88
pipe networks
　cleaning 76–84
　design 39–46
　health checklists 65–6
　maintenance 75–9
　non-aggressive cleaning 76, 77–8, 79–84
　operation 39–46
　pathogenic microorganisms 88
　survey procedures 75–9
planning
　mains cleaning programs 78–9
　mixing conditions 53–4
point-of-delivery 59–65
point-of-entry 9–11
point-of-use 9–11
population sizes, animals 106–8
potable water 60–2, 90–1
powdered carbon 31–2
power supplies 52
pressure
　chlorination stations 52
　jetting 73, 76
　maintenance and survey procedures 70
　piped network hydraulics 40, 41
　potable water systems 60–2
　relief valves 44–5
　surges 44–5
preventing bacterial proliferation 21–30
principles of microbial monitoring 13–14
prioritizing risks 128–30
process validation monitoring 131, 132, 134–5
property types 63–4
protozoan parasites 8, 9
Pseudomonas 6–7
pump capacity 52
pumping 49
pumps 42–3, 44–5
pyrethroids 114–15

quality objectives 21–30

Rairangpur, Orisa, India 88
RDOC *see* refractory dissolved organic carbon
record keeping 50, 135–6
reduced pressure zone assemblies (RPZA) 63

Index

refractory dissolved organic carbon (RDOC) 27–8
regulations and microbiological parameters 12–13
relay stations 33, 50–2, 94
remedial measures, animal infestations 112–18
renovation works 87, 94
repair works 87–99
residence time 49
residual disinfectant *see* disinfectant residuals
restricted operations 90–1
reviewing water safety plans 133
risks
  assessments
    construction/repair works 96–7
    semiquantitative 129
    service reservoirs 49–50
    water safety plans 125–7
  characterization 125–30
  construction/repair works 82, 94, 96–7
  management 121–36
  prioritizing 128–30
  ranking 128–30
  repair works 87–9
  service reservoirs 49–50
  water safety plans 125–7
robotic cleaning equipment 73
roundworms 116
routine inspections/sampling 14, 15
RPZA *see* reduced pressure zone assemblies

Salmonella 110–11
sampling
  animal occurrences 103–4
  construction/repair works 97
  microbial monitoring 14
  microbial safety 2–3
  service reservoirs 50
  source mixing conditions 54–5
sand filters 31
sanitary significance
  backflow/cross-connections 59–60
  maintenance/survey procedures 70–1, 75–6
sanitary surveys
  controlling microorganisms 11
  frequency 73
  microbial monitoring principles 14
  water safety plans 127–8, 129
scale 29–30, 128
Scandinavia 3–4
Schistosoma 109
seals 70
security of sites 49
sediments 8, 70
semiquantitative risk assessments 129
septic tanks 75
service reservoirs
  animal infestations 118
  animal occurrences 105
  design/operation 46–50, 66
  maintenance/survey procedures 70–5, 84
sewage systems 61
shape of service reservoirs 47–8
Shigella 110–11
shrimps 115–16
significance
  backflow/cross-connections 59–60
  maintenance/survey procedures 70–1, 75–6
  metazoan animals 108–12
site security 49
siting
  chlorination stations 51
  pipes 59, 66–7
slaters 115
slug flows 83
small community-managed systems 97–8
snails 116
sodium hypochlorite 94
software 44–5, 54
source mixing conditions 53–6
source protection 5

South America 4
stagnation 9, 46
standard forms 128
State of Georgia, USA 126
stop taps 64–5
stratification 49
supply losses 49
supporting programmes 135
surge shafts 44–5
surges 44–5, 70–1
survey procedures 69–85
swabbing
  animal infestations 113
  pipe network cleaning 76, 79, 80, 81–2
switching pumps 44–5
system assessments 122
system-specific validation 135
systematic unidirectional flushing 112–13, 114–15

tanks
  break 62, 64
  maintenance/survey procedures 70–4, 75, 84
telemetry 52, 133
temperature 20, 56
testing 54, 56, 64–5
thermotolerant coliforms 12–13, 15
THMs *see* trihalomethanes
TOC *see* total organic carbon
total coliform counts 12, 32
total organic carbon (TOC) 28, 32
training 97–8
treated water, microbial quality 19–34
treatment works
  animal infestations 104–5, 117–18
  microbiology 5–6
trihalomethanes (THMs) 22, 23
trophic interactions 107
trunk mains 43
turbidity 26

UK *see* United Kingdom

ultrafiltration 31–2
underground pipe rigs 95–6
unidirectional flushing 112–13, 114–15
United Kingdom (UK)
  animal occurrences 102
  Bristol 98
  Clitheroe Lancashire 10
  construction/repair works 95–6
  particulate content 26
  waterborne disease 3
United States of America (USA)
  Arizona 61
  construction/repair works 96
  Georgia 126
  Massachusetts 41
  Missouri 4–5
  Pierce County, Washington State 75
  waterborne disease 3
urban water safety plans 128
USA *see* United States of America
Uzbekistan 4

valve chambers 43
valves 44–5, 74–5
verification monitoring 131, 132, 133–5
Vibrio cholerae 4
viruses
  animal associations 110–11
  enteric 9
  microbiology 8, 9
  Norwalk 75, 126
volumetric dosing 52

washout valves 42
water
  composition changes 56
  depth 47
  fleas 8, 106, 108–9, 117
  purification devices 9–11
  quality
    deterioration 32
    treated water microbial 30

Index

safety plans 3, 122–36
usage devices 9
waterborne disease 3–15
 see also individual diseases
WHO Pesticide Evaluation Scheme (WHOPES) 114–15
WHOPES *see* WHO Pesticide Evaluation Scheme
working practice guidelines 89–90

wormlike organisms 116
worms
 flat 109
 guinea worm 8, 108
 oligochaete worms 113, 115, 116
 remedial measures 113, 116
 roundworms 116

zoning networks 57–8, 66